Epidemiology of HIV

in Mwanza Region, Tanzania

Academisch proefschrift
ter verkrijging van de graad van doctor
aan de Universiteit van Amsterdam,
op gezag van de Rector Magnificus prof. dr P.W.M. de Meijer,
ten overstaan van een door het college van dekanen ingestelde
commissie in het openbaar te verdedigen in de Aula der Universiteit
(Oude Lutherse Kerk, ingang Singel 411, hoek Spui),
op donderdag 20 oktober 1994 te 15.00 uur

door

Martinus Willem Borgdorff
geboren te Gorinchem

Promotiecommissie

Promotores	Prof dr R A Coutinho
	Prof dr A S Muller
Leden	Prof dr J Huisman, Prof dr J van der Noordaa,
	Prof dr J P Tijssen, dr C Varkevisser
Faculteit	Faculteit der Geneeskunde

The research described in this thesis was carried out in the Tanzania-Netherlands Research Project on AIDS and HIV Infection in Mwanza Region, a collaborative project of the National Institute for Medical Research Mwanza, Regional Medical Office Mwanza, Bugando Medical Centre, Royal Tropical Institute Amsterdam, and the Institute for International Health of Nijmegen University.

Research for this publication was financed by the Netherlands' Ministry for Development Cooperation, Section for Research and Technology, P.O. Box 20061, 2500 EB, The Hague, as part of the Tanzania-Netherlands Research Project on AIDS and HIV Infection in Mwanza Region. Publication was financially supported by the Stichting AIDS Research Amsterdam and the Stichting Sarphati.

CIP-DATA KONINKLIJKE BIBLIOTHEEK, DEN HAAG

Borgdorff, Martinus Willem

Epidemiology of HIV-infection in Mwanza Region, Tanzania / Martinus Willem Borgdorff. - Amsterdam : Royal Tropical Institute
Thesis Universiteit van Amsterdam. - With ref.
ISBN 90-6832-094-7
NUGI 742
Subject headings: AIDS ; Tanzania.

© 1994 Royal Tropical Institute - Amsterdam
Cover design: Freek Thielsch – Amsterdam
Cartography: J. ter Haar – Hoofddorp
Printer: Krips Repro – Meppel

ISBN 90 6832 094 7
NUGI 742

Table of contents

I

Introduction

Human immunodeficiency virus (HIV) infection is a major public health problem in Africa not only because of its medical consequences, including AIDS, but also because of its damaging social and economic implications [1]. Of the two types of HIV present in Africa, type 1 (HIV-1) is much more prevalent and probably also more virulent [2,3]. As to date in Tanzania all HIV is of type 1, the review below is restricted to HIV-1.

How commonly do HIV infection and AIDS occur in Africa?

Notified AIDS cases
By June 1993, 718,894 cases of AIDS had been notified to the World Health Organization (WHO) from all over the world [4]. Of these cases, 247/577 (34%) were reported from Africa, in which 12% of the world population lives. Of all cases of AIDS in Africa notified by June 1993, 49% were from Tanzania, Uganda, Kenya, Rwanda, and Burundi (in descending order for the absolute number of cases) [4], while only 13% (81/642 million) of Africa's total population lives there [5].

AIDS notification is incomplete, particularly in most developing countries [6,7]. This is due to the following factors:

- Not all AIDS cases are diagnosed, particularly in areas where health facilities are limited in number and quality and where patients may prefer alternative sources of health care [7-10].
- Not all diagnosed cases may be notified by the health service providers to the Ministry of Health or by the Ministry to WHO because of deficient administration or for political reasons [7,8,10].

The degree of incompleteness is likely to vary between different countries and areas and also over time.

Differences in the AIDS case definition between countries and over time are another complication when making comparisons [7,10,11], although its effect is relatively small compared with the incompleteness of reporting [7]. Because of the limited availability of laboratory facilities in Africa a clinical AIDS case definition [12] has been widely used with minor modifications in various countries [7,9,10,13,14]. A major change in this definition, including the requirement of a positive HIV test, has been applied in Ivory Coast [13].

Because AIDS is a late consequence of HIV infection, making use of notified AIDS cases is unsuitable for the detection of recent changes in HIV prevalence [7,11,15]. However, the advantage of using AIDS notification is that the method is cheap and

Figure 1. Map of the United Republic of Tanzania

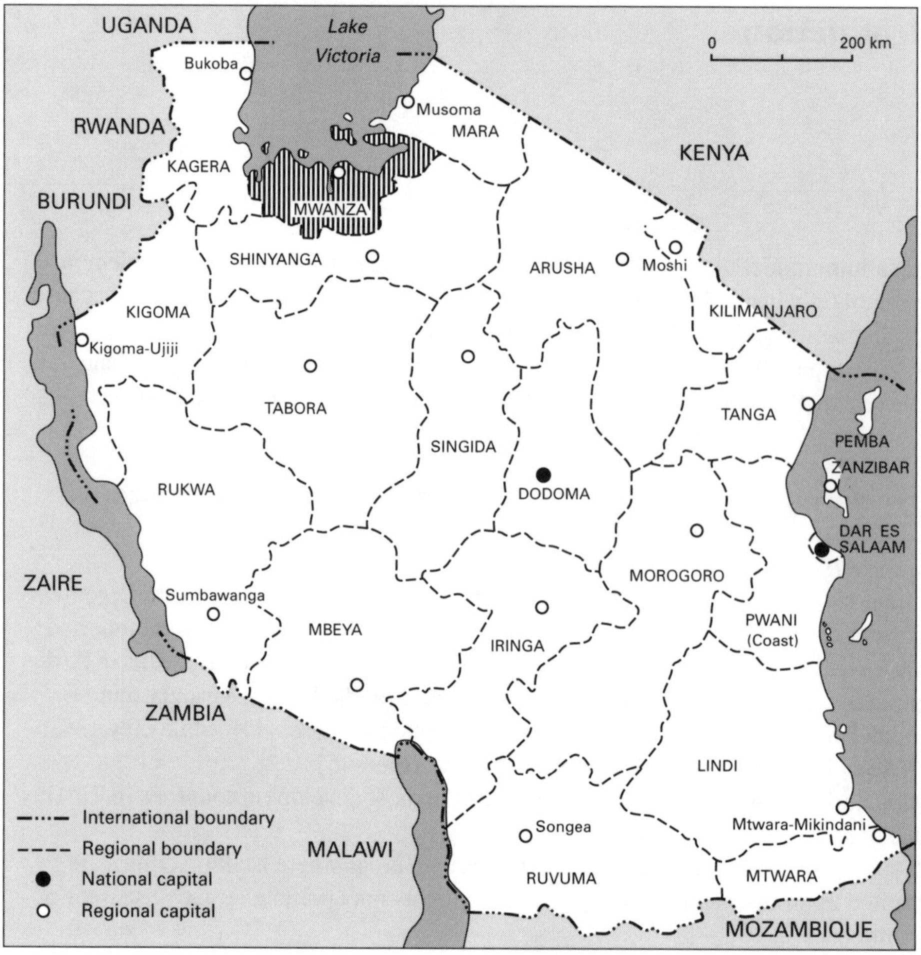

almost universally applied, and that it provides an indicator to assess the medical and financial burden of the AIDS epidemic [7,9,13].

Prevalence of HIV-1 infection
Because of the limitations in AIDS notification, monitoring HIV prevalence in selected groups such as blood donors or pregnant women has been advocated [15,16], with a preference being expressed for unlinked anonymous testing in order to avoid participation bias within the selected groups [7,16–20]. HIV prevalence has been monitored successfully in pregnant women or newborn babies in developed countries [21–27], and also in developing countries [28,29]. The National AIDS Control Programme of Tanzania monitors HIV prevalence in blood donors, who are mostly relatives of blood recipients, as its most important source of information on the size of the HIV epidemic [30].

Information on HIV-1 prevalence in selected groups may be difficult to interpret as the degree of selection bias is unknown [31]. However, as these groups are selected for reasons of convenience, it is relatively cheap and easy to follow trends over time. The validity of extrapolating trends in such sentinel groups to the general population is uncertain and may vary from one area to another as well as over time.

Population surveys, if carried out well, may provide the least biased estimate of HIV-1 prevalence, provided participation bias can be minimized [7]. However, very few general population surveys have been carried out, partly because of their cost and partly because in many countries a large number of people would refuse to participate in such surveys. To date in Tanzania, general population surveys have been published from two regions: Kagera [32] and Mwanza [33] (see Chapter 3). One of their uses has been to assess the validity of data obtained from sentinel surveillance [31] (see Chapter 4). In Mwanza Region HIV-1 prevalence in blood donors, who were relatives of the blood recipients, was close to that in the general population, provided the data were standardized for urban/non-urban location, age and sex [31] (see Chapter 4).

WHO estimated that by the end of 1992 at least 8 million people in Africa were infected with HIV, most of them with type 1 [34]. With a total population of 642 million [5], this is a crude prevalence rate of 1.2%. For comparison, WHO's estimate for Europe was 0.5 million infected people [34], giving a crude prevalence rate of 0.1%. Because the demographic structure in Africa is different from Europe, with a smaller proportion of the population being aged 15 to 64 years (52% in Africa versus 67% in Europe [5]) these crude prevalence rates underestimate the differences in the rates in the adult population. Furthermore, the difference in HIV prevalence rates in Africa and Europe is still growing [34].

Within Africa HIV-1 infection is not evenly distributed: it is at present much more common in East and Central than in West Africa [2,35,36]. In Tanzania, the National AIDS Control Programme estimated the total number of HIV-1-infected individuals to be 750,000 in 1990 [30], 725,000 of whom were aged 15 years and above. From a total population of 28 million [5], this gives a crude prevalence rate of 3% in the total population and of 5% in adults. Within Tanzania the most affected areas are thought to be Kagera Region in the northwest, Mbeya, Rukwa and Iringa in the Southern Highlands, Dar es Salaam, the capital and Tanga, at the coast [30] (See Figure 1, Map of Tanzania). Mwanza Region, in which the studies presented in the next chapters took place, ranks close to the median regarding the number of notified AIDS cases and HIV prevalence in blood donors [30]. While the former depends heavily on the completeness of reporting and is therefore not easy to interpret, HIV prevalence in blood donors is a more robust measure, as incomplete reporting affects the numerator and denominator to a similar degree.

Incidence of HIV-1 infection in adults
Measuring the incidence of HIV infection is desirable to monitor the speed at which the epidemic spreads in a particular location. In addition, when studies are planned to evaluate the efficacy of interventions to reduce HIV transmission, for instance through condom promotion, control of sexually transmitted diseases (STD) or immunization, a reasonable estimate of the incidence of HIV infection is required for the determination

of the size of the sample needed for the study [37]. Published literature on the incidence of HIV-1 infection in Africa is limited [2], probably because it can only be
measured in difficult and costly longitudinal studies [38]. An overview of published
HIV-1 incidence studies in Africa is given in Table 1. Of the 17 studies, 9 took place in
the general population [39–41] or in groups with HIV prevalences comparable to the
general population: workers at a factory and a hospital [42–44], police officers [45] and
antenatal clinic attenders [46,47]. The other half of the surveys concerned high-risk
groups such as prostitutes [48–52], STD clinic attenders [53] and spouses of HIV infected
people [54,55]. As might be expected, the incidence was lowest in general population
groups and much higher in risk groups.

In a general population cohort in Tanzania, HIV-1 incidence was 0.8 per 100 person-
years in rural and 4.8 in urban areas [39]. In two rural areas in Uganda the annual
incidence was 2.1% for those aged 13 years and above in one study [40] and 1.1% in
another [41]. In Kinshasa hospital workers the incidence was 1–2% [42,43]. In Mwanza,
incidence in urban factory workers was similar at 1.2% per year [44] (see Chapter 9).
In police officers in Guinea-Bissau, the incidence was 0.8% per year in a population
with a prevalence at intake of 0.4% [45]. In women recruited at antenatal clinics in the
capital cities of Rwanda and Zambia the incidence was 3% to 4% [46,47]. Among
spouses of HIV-1 infected people in Rwanda and Zaire, the incidence was 2% to 6% in
the presence of an effective counselling programme [54,55]. The prevalence and
incidence of HIV-1 were still low in prostitutes in Somalia in 1988 [52], but high rates
of approximately 10% were found among prostitutes in Kinshasa and Yaounde [49,50],
while extremely high rates were documented in selected prostitute groups and STD
clinic attenders in Nairobi [48,51,53].

Risk factors for HIV-1 infection in Africa

Whereas HIV-1 infection in developed countries is primarily transmitted through
homosexual intercourse and needle sharing among intravenous drug users, the main
transmission route in Africa is heterosexual intercourse [35,56–63]. In addition, transmission occurs through blood transfusions and from mother to child, and – probably
much less – through contaminated injections [35,58,62,64,65].

Potential risk factors for heterosexual HIV-1 transmission have been identified in a
large number of studies. New cases of HIV-1 infection are most likely to occur in
individuals who have sexual intercourse with multiple partners [2,32,33,58,60,62,
63,66–74] or whose sexual partners have multiple partners [52,70,75–78], without
using condoms [46,48,54,71,79–89] in an environment where HIV-1 is highly prevalent
[60,61,71]. Transmission has been shown to be more likely if the infected partner has a
high viral load, such as in advanced HIV disease and AIDS [61,83,84,87,88,90–93].

Other potential risk factors for HIV infection (perhaps partly through an association
with risk behaviour and risk environment) have been identified as follows: other STDs,
sexual techniques, male circumcision, sex, age, urban/rural residence, mobility and
socioeconomic status. These risk factors are discussed in more detail below.

Table I.   Overview of results of studies on the incidence of HIV-I in Africa

Country	Year	Sex	Cohort size	Person-years	Sero conv (Nr)	Incid. rate (/100 pyr)	Annual rate of lost to follow up	Reference
General population								
Tanzania	1987-89	M+F	1316	2406	33	1.4	19%	(39)
Uganda	1989-90	M+F	1037	978	21	2.1	25%	(40)
Uganda	1989-91	M+F	5251	1216	13	1.1	30%	(41)
Occupational cohorts								
Zaire	1984-85	M+F	749	±405	3	0.7	32%	(42)
Zaire	1984-86	M+F	1905	3748	62	1.7	8%	(43)
Tanzania	1991-93	M+F	1567	1366	17	1.2	14%	(44)
Guinea-Bissau	1991-92	M+F	797	687	5	0.8	44%	(45)
Antenatal clinic attenders								
Zambia	1987-88	F	1720	±634	16	3.0	63%	(47).
Rwanda	1986-88	F	1057	n/a	n/a	4.1 }	4%	(46)
Rwanda	1988-90	F	970	n/a	n/a	3.0 }		
Spouses of HIV infected people								
Rwanda	1988-91	M	23	53	2	3.8 }	8%	(54)
		F	30	63	6	6.4 }		
Zaire	1988-89	M	69	90	4	4.4 }	6%	(55)
		F	80	100	2	2.0 }		
Prostitutes								
Kenya	1985-87	F	124	182	83	45.5	37%	(48)
Somalia	1988	F	155	41	1	2	>50%	(52)
Zaire	1988-	F	431	778	76	9.8	n/a	(49)
Kenya	1987-90	F	138	149	47	31.5	15%	(51)
Cameroon	1989-90	F	273	184	19	10.4	8%	(50)
STD clinic attenders								
Kenya	1986-87	M	293	79	24	30	>21%	(53)

Note: If parameters were not reported in the papers concerned, an estimate was made from other data presented. If such an estimate was not possible, n/a (not available) is indicated. Abstracts from 1991 and earlier have been excluded from this overview.

Other sexually transmitted diseases. Other sexually transmitted diseases, in particular genital ulcer disease, have been shown to be associated with HIV infection [38,52,61–63, 66,67,69,71,74–76,78,84,90,94–103]. This association is partly due to confounding as both HIV and other STDs are a consequence of high-risk sexual behaviour [98,104]. As HIV-1 infection is probably associated with an increased incidence of genital ulcers [98], this provides an alternative explanation for their association in cross-sectional studies. However, prospective studies in extremely high-risk populations have confirmed that genital ulcers [53,98] and genital discharge (gonorrhoea, chlamydia and perhaps trichomonas) [49] may facilitate HIV transmission. In the latter study the population attributable risk of genital discharge was found to be considerably higher than that of genital ulcer [49].

In a study in Rwanda, 32% of urban women were found to be infected with HIV [75]. Although reported STD in the past 5 years was the risk factor showing the strongest association with HIV, only 30% of HIV-1 infected women reported this risk factor. This suggests that at the community level the impact of STD control on HIV transmission might be limited.

Sexual techniques. There is limited evidence, mainly from developed countries, on the risk of various sexual techniques for heterosexual transmission. An increased risk of male to female transmission has been shown to be associated with anal intercourse [89,90,92,93] and may be associated with vaginal intercourse during the menstrual period [75]. Female to male transmission has been shown to be associated with sexual intercourse during the menstrual period [93].

Male circumcision. Conflicting evidence exists on the association between circum- cision and HIV infection. A strong protective effect of circumcision was suggested by studies among STD clinic attenders in Nairobi and Abidjan [53,76,78,95,105]. This association was supported by studies comparing populations rather than individuals [106–108]. However, no association was found in studies in Rwanda [75,101,109]. In Mwanza no association was found in a population survey [33] (see Chapter 3), but a protective effect was suggested in the factory cohort study [110] (see Chapter 7). In this cohort, circumcision was associated with higher levels of socioeconomic status and condom use, which may have caused confounding in some of the above studies.

Cervical ectopy; bleeding after sexual intercourse. In one study from Nairobi, cervical ectopy was associated with HIV infection in univariate analysis and after adjustment for age, pregnancy, and oral contraceptive use [112]. In some studies non-menstrual blood loss after sexual intercourse (of unspecified causes) was associated with risk of HIV infection in women [75,89].

Contraceptive use. There is evidence that HIV can not pass through latex condoms [79], and that condoms protect against other sexually transmitted diseases [80,88]. Epidemiological evidence suggests that partners of discordant couples (in which one partner is HIV-infected and the other is not) can reduce their risk of HIV infection by using condoms [54,80,81–84]. In prostitutes condom use is associated with a lower prevalence [71,85] and incidence [86] of HIV infection. A counselling and condom promotion programme among women of child-bearing age in Rwanda contributed towards an increased use of condoms and a reduction in HIV incidence [46]. Therefore, it is clear that condom use reduces HIV transmission.

The effect of the use of nonoxynol-9 spermicides in preventing HIV transmission is not clear [113,114]. In a prospective study in Cameroon, a strong protective effect was demonstrated [50], but in a randomized, placebo-controlled trial in Nairobi, HIV infection tended to occur more frequently in the nonoxynol-9 sponge users (odds ratio 1.6, 95% confidence interval 0.8–2.8) [51]. In the latter study nonoxynol-9 use was associated with a higher incidence of genital ulcers and a reduced incidence of gonococcal cervical infection [51]. A reduced incidence of gonorrhoeal and chlamydial cervical infections was demonstrated in another randomised, controlled trial [115]. Nonoxynol-9 use is commonly associated with vaginal irritation [50,51,115].

The effect of oral contraceptives is also not clear. In Nairobi use of oral contraceptives was associated with an increased HIV-1 prevalence [97] and incidence [50]. In Rwanda oral contraceptive use was reported more frequently in HIV-infected couples than in non-infected couples [109]. No association was found between oral contraceptive use and the prevalence or incidence of HIV infection among prostitutes in Zaire [49,71], while in Italy oral contraceptives were associated with a reduced prevalence of HIV in heterosexual partners of HIV-infected men [84].

There are several limitations in these observations on the association between HIV and oral contraceptive use. A general limitation is that contraceptive use is only one aspect of sexual behaviour, and is likely to be associated with other aspects such as sexual partner change, for which complete control is impossible to achieve in studies [104]. A practical limitation in planning further studies is the generally low contraceptive use in Africa. Experimental studies with random allocation to various contraceptive methods would provide more convincing evidence but may be impossible for practical and ethical reasons.

In Italy use of an intra-uterine contraceptive device (IUD) was associated with an increased HIV prevalence in women [84]. From Africa no reports on an association were found.

Genetic factors. There is some evidence from a cohort study among prostitutes in Nairobi that those with major histocompatability complex (MHC) class I alleles Aw28 and Bw70 have a reduced risk of HIV seroconversion, while those with Aw19 have an increased risk [116]. This association might be due to differences in susceptibility, which itself might be due to genetically determined differences in the operating mechanisms of the immune system.

Sex. In East Africa HIV-1 infection is more common among women than men, in particular in urban areas, with a ratio of sex-specific prevalence (F/M) between 1 and 2 [32,33,74,117–119]. This might be partly explained by the effect of participation bias [117,120]. If a real difference exists, it might be due to a greater efficiency of male-female than of female-male transmission [91,93,117,121] or a longer incubation period in women, which in turn may be partly due to women becoming infected at a younger age [117]. Finally, it has been suggested that the stage of the epidemic might play a role: in the early stages a small group of prostitutes might infect a large group of men, whereas later this large group of men would infect an even larger group of other women. As neither the efficiency of female-male and male-female transmission nor the natural history of HIV-1 infection in Africa have been adequately studied, these explanations remain largely speculative.

Age. Age groups with highest HIV-1 and AIDS prevalence are 15–34 years among women and 25–44 years among men [10,30,33,35,57,58,63,74,75,117–119]. The age specific prevalence is probably determined largely by age specific incidence in the early stages of the epidemic; in later stages HIV-1 associated mortality is another determinant.

Residence. HIV-1 infection has been found to be strongly associated with urban residence [32,33,36,58,62,73,74,118,119]. This may be due to an earlier introduction of HIV-1 in urban areas, but may in addition be due to risk behaviour being more pronounced there [74,122]. The latter explanation is supported by other observations, for instance that other STDs occur more frequently in urban areas [33,36,98,119].

Mobility. Travelling may be a risk factor for HIV infection [32,33,74,78,94,123,124], for which there are two obvious explanations. Those travelling to an area with a high HIV prevalence are at an increased risk compared with those staying at home [32,74, 123,124]. In addition, travel may be associated with acquiring high-risk sexual partners in bars and guesthouses on the way [32,94,124]. This latter explanation may be true in particular for truck drivers, who have been identified as a high-risk group in East Africa [94,125].

Socioeconomic status: education, income. HIV-1 infection and AIDS in Africa have been reported in some studies to be associated with higher levels of education and income [57,58,74,75,103], but the opposite was found by others [76,96,123]. In sexual behaviour surveys it has been observed that risk behaviour was more common among those with a higher level of education in a number of countries, but not in all [122]. Those with a higher level of income are in a position to acquire sexual favours in exchange for material favours; this would put them at higher risk, unless change of behaviour takes place once this risk has been recognized. It has also been suggested that in the early stages of the epidemic in a particular region those of higher socioeconomic status may be more likely to travel and acquire the infection elsewhere; once HIV has been introduced in a site it may spread to all strata of society [123]. Eventually it might affect mostly those in lower socioeconomic strata, as appears to be the case in the United States [126–129] because preventive programmes are least successful there.

Religion. Various religions have different rules on the types of permitted sexual behaviour. For instance, some religions are against condom use, others are not; some allow polygamy, others do not. These rules may vary in strictness in their content and control of their application. One might therefore expect to find an association between religion and risk for HIV infection. Few papers have reported on religion as a risk factor for HIV-1 [74,75,130,131]. Only one study [130,131] from Africa showed an association between (non-Muslim) religion and risk for HIV infection, which the authors explained by the negative association between HIV and circumcision on the one hand and religion and circumcision on the other. In Mwanza, no association was found between risk behaviour and religion in the factory cohort study [111] (see Chapter 8).

Interventions to reduce heterosexual HIV-1 transmission

From the information on risk factors, it is obvious that there are several interventions which may be expected to reduce heterosexual HIV-1 transmission. These include ones aimed at reducing the rate of sexual partner change and increasing the use of condoms, and the early and adequate treatment of STDs [80,132–134,135]. Preventive interventions aiming at reducing parenteral HIV-1 transmission, in particular by blood transfusion [1,64,134], and perinatal transmission [1,134] will not be discussed here.

The heterosexual population can be subdivided according to the level of risk: first priority should be given to those at highest risk, called the core group [136] or primary risk group [137]. This group comprises those who frequently change sexual partners, including prostitutes and their clients. The next target for attention is the secondary risk group, comprising sexual partners of those in the primary risk group. A third target group consists of adolescents, even those presently at low risk because they can be expected to be at high risk in the near future [137]. Others have suggested using the term high-risk situation instead of high-risk group or behaviour, in order to emphasize the social, economic and political setting instead of just the characteristics of the individuals concerned [138].

WHO proposes that action to change sexual behaviour should have three components: information and education, backed up by health and social services, and a supportive environment [1]. Information and education should be forthright and clear. Those who have multiple sexual partners, or who are unsure of the infection status of their partner, need to know that they can reduce the risk of HIV infection by avoiding penetrative sex or by using latex condoms consistently and correctly. Parents, teachers, and traditional, religious and other community leaders have an important role to play in reinforcing traditional health-promoting values and practices. Experience also points to the importance of peer education, in which a person who enjoys the trust of his or her peers brings prevention messages and skills to them, rather than an educator from outside the peer group [1].

Condom promotion has been successful with the peer education approach, and by using social marketing, community-based distribution or a mixture of these [80,134, 137]. Major problems encountered are those associated with a bad image of condoms, with supply and logistics, and the high cost of consistent condom use. The possibilities of a female condom are being explored: so far its high cost is a major barrier.

Health and social services are extremely important for the early detection and treatment of STDs. An outline of major issues in planning and implementing STD control is given by Piot and Hira [139]. Important issues are treatment seeking behaviour, early and simple diagnosis, quality of laboratory services, an adequate drug supply system, locally valid and simple STD treatment guidelines, and training of health workers [134,139]. STD management guidelines have been developed by WHO [140]. Health and social services can also provide AIDS education, counselling, and voluntary HIV testing. For instance, confidential HIV testing and counselling were shown to be effective in increasing condom use and reducing HIV seroconversion in discordant couples in Rwanda and Zaire [46,54,55].

A supportive environment is vital because of the importance of the norms of peers and community in regulating the behaviour of individuals. The adoption, readoption or retention of protective social norms such as mutual fidelity, moral responsibility for not harming others, and appropriate use of condoms may need to be encouraged. In addition, legal and other barriers may need to be removed which hinder the dissemination of frank and informative messages, or restrain people from acting on those messages. A supportive environment is one that does not stigmatize or discriminate against people with HIV or AIDS. Special emphasis needs to be given to the position of women. Women run considerable risks of becoming HIV infected, but frequently lack the means to protect themselves, because of illiteracy, poverty, or insufficient say in their own and their partners' sexual decision making [1].

Given the broad social and economic consequences of the AIDS epidemic, its control should be multisectoral. It should also involve as much as possible the efforts of non-government organizations, because of their strong links to individuals and communities [1].

A supportive environment is one that also provides care for people with HIV or AIDS. This care includes counselling (so is partly preventive) and provision of medical care. Provision of appropriate counselling and medical care depends partly on knowledge of the natural history of HIV-1 infection, which is discussed in more detail in the next section.

Natural history of HIV-1 infection in adults in Africa

Information on the natural history of HIV-1 infection in adults in Africa is still very limited [141]. Aspects of interest include the incubation period (between acquiring HIV-1 infection and developing AIDS) and the time period from infection to death, the proportion of people dying before developing AIDS, risk factors for progression to disease and death, simple laboratory markers for progression, the incidence and clinical presentation of diseases associated with HIV-1 infection, and appropriate treatment for HIV associated diseases within the constraints posed by limited diagnostic facilities and limited funds for drugs.

Incubation period and time period from infection to death
In the USA and Europe the incubation period between acquiring HIV-1 infection and developing AIDS has been determined to have a median of 7 to 10 years in homosexual men, haemophiliacs, and blood transfusion recipients [142–149]. In intravenous drug abusers the incubation period was found to be similar [150]. However, in the latter group a sizable proportion of deaths may occur in HIV-1 infected people who have not yet developed AIDS [151–153] (e.g. 13/41=32% [153]). These results were based on a less inclusive AIDS case definition than the one recently adopted by the Centers for Disease Control in 1992 for the USA [154], which will lead to a much shorter incubation period [155–158].

In Africa a clinical case definition of AIDS with limited sensitivity and specificity is used [9,11,12,159–161]. For this reason, and because there may be a sizeable mortality in HIV-infected individuals before the development of AIDS, it has been suggested that it may be more informative to study mortality than the incidence of AIDS [162].

In Africa no cohorts have been followed for long enough to make a direct measurement of the incubation period or of the period from infection to death. By breaking up these periods into stages and calculating the probability of moving from one stage to the next (or back to the previous stage), the period from infection to death has been estimated through a mathematical model developed in Nairobi [163]. This model was based on data from the follow-up of a cohort of prostitutes and indicated that the period between infection and the development of symptoms in this cohort might be shorter than that in homosexuals in the USA and Europe [163]. The mean period from infection to death was estimated at 9 to 12 years, which would be comparable to results in Europe and the USA. However, only 4 deaths were observed, so these estimates have a wide margin of uncertainty. In Rwanda 14/27 (52%) prostitutes had died within 8 years after having been found to be HIV infected [164]; another 2 were lost to follow up. The time of seroconversion in this group was not known.

The evidence is insufficient to decide whether or not the period from infection to death in Africa is shorter than in developed countries. Direct measurement of mortality rates in a cohort in Africa with a long period of follow-up is therefore desirable. Because of the lengthy period from infection to death, results will take a long time to be obtained. However, preliminary ones might be estimated by using the staging system of HIV infection and disease developed by WHO [165–168]. Once such a study has achieved a sufficient duration, its results may then be used to validate the WHO staging system by providing information on the prognosis of various stages in Africa [167].

HIV-1-associated mortality
HIV infection has been shown to contribute substantially to mortality in hospitals in Africa [169–176]. An obvious limitation of these studies is their selection bias, as in Africa many people die at home.

In an occupational cohort study in Zaire, 35 (21.5%) out of 163 factory and office workers who died were found to have had AIDS, making AIDS the most common cause of death [103]. HIV-1 prevalence in these factory and office workers was 3% and 6% respectively [103]. In women followed up post-partum in Zaire, 29 deaths occurred in approximately 710 person-years of follow-up in HIV-1-infected women (4 per 100), and none in 930 person-years of follow-up in non-HIV-1-infected women [177]. In a prospective cohort study in Rwanda, mortality was compared between HIV-1-infected and non-HIV-1-infected women [162]. The HIV-1 prevalence in this representative sample of urban women of child-bearing age was 33%. Mortality after 24 months in the two groups was 7% in those with and 0.3% in those without HIV infection, giving a relative risk of 23. Of all deaths 90% occurred in HIV-infected individuals. In two community-based studies in Uganda, similar mortality rates were observed: in the age group 13 years and above (male and female combined) mortality was 10.3/100 person-years (31 deaths) in HIV-1 seropositives and 0.8/100 person-years (29 deaths) in HIV-1 seronegatives (41); in the other study these rates were 5.2% (20 deaths) and 0.7% (30 deaths), respectively [178]. After two years of follow-up in Mwanza among factory workers with a prevalence of HIV-1 infection of 12%, the crude mortality rate was 4.9% (14 deaths) in HIV-1-infected individuals and 0.3% (3 deaths) in non-HIV-1-infected individuals, giving an age- and sex-adjusted relative risk of death of 12.9; 62% of deaths were attributable to HIV-1 infection [44] (see Chapter 9). Although these data are limited, it seems reasonable to conclude that HIV-1 has a major impact on mortality in adults in Africa, as has been predicted by a variety of mathematical models [8,179–181].

In developed countries an elaborate literature exists on predictors of HIV-1 disease progression among homosexuals, haemophiliacs, and intravenous drug users, recently summarized by Mientjes [182]. These include demographic and behavioural factors such as older age [143,150,183–186], high rate of sexual partner change [187,188], having other STDs before or after seroconversion [187], and having had sexual intercourse with a person with AIDS [189,190]; clinical indicators such as primary HIV infection with symptoms for more than 14 days [182,190] and thereafter the occurrence of symptoms such as fever, night sweats, fatigue, weight loss, dyspnoea, pneumonia, endocarditis, tuberculosis, chronic diarrhoea, oral thrush or herpes zoster [147,153,188, 189,191–194]; laboratory markers such as low CD4 count [147,153,184,185,188–192, 194–199], low CD4 percent [153,196,198], low CD4/CD8 ratio [188,194], rate of decline of CD4 count [192,200] or CD4 percent [198], high β_2-microglobulin [147,185,194–197, 201], high neopterin [147,185,191,195,201], high IgG and IgA [185,188,196,202], presence of HIV p24 core antigen [147,185,189,190,194–197,201], low titre of core antibody [185,189,190,195], presence of fast-replicating, syncytium-inducing HIV-1 [199,200,202–205], and possibly the presence of certain HLA haplotypes [206,207]. Most of these predictors reflect the development of immunodeficiency in the patient in the course of HIV-1 infection; some may be associated with virulence of the virus [205]; while the presence of certain HLA haplotypes may reflect genetically determined susceptibility or immune response.

Only a few publications appear to be available on predictors of progression of HIV-1 disease in Africa, as laboratory facilities are usually limited and follow-up studies rare. That laboratory predictors in Africa are not necessarily identical to those in Europe is illustrated by a comparative study on HIV antigenaemia and HIV core antibodies, which showed marked differences between European and African individuals [208]. β_2-Microglobulin was shown in a small study in Dar es Salaam to be a good predictor for HIV-associated death [209]. In the Gambia clinical predictors for mortality in a group of HIV-1- and HIV-2-infected hospital attenders were Karnofsky score and diagnosis of AIDS [210]. Laboratory predictors were $\log_e$ serum neopterin level, CD4 cell count and $\log_e$ serum β_2-microglobulin. In univariate analysis CD4 percentage and total lymphocyte count were also strong predictors, but in the multivariate model they added no predictive power after including the other three laboratory variables.

In a prospective cohort study in Rwanda, the following predictors of mortality were identified [162]: body mass index of 21 kg/m^2 or less (relative hazard 2.3), low income (relative hazard 2.3), erythrocyte sedimentation rate more than 60 mm/hr (relative hazard 4.9), chronic diarrhoea (relative hazard 2.6), history of herpes zoster (relative hazard 5.3), and oral candidiasis (relative hazard 7.3). If out of five predictors (income was excluded) three or more were present, mortality was 33% after two years; mortality rates after two years for those with two, one, or no predictors were 14%, 5%, and 0%, respectively. The great advantage of the markers used in this study is that they can be employed widely in Africa, as opposed to CD4 counts, which can only be carried out in a few centres. However, the validation of these markers in other settings is required. Other relatively simple markers to be evaluated more widely might be serum β_2-microglobulin, serum albumin [193], anaemia [186] and triglyceride levels [211].

HIV-1-associated morbidity
In a review Colebunders and Latif summarize the clinical manifestations of HIV-1 infection in adults in Africa [141]. These include: dermatological manifestations such as generalized papular pruritic eruption, herpes zoster, hypersensitivity reactions and herpes simplex infection; oral manifestations such as oral candidiasis, ulcero-necrotic gingivitis, oral Kaposi sarcoma lesions and aphthous ulcers; weight loss; fever associated with a variety of infections (e.g. *M. tuberculosis, Cryptococcus neoformans*, and *Salmonella septicaemia*) or malignancies (eg non-Hodgkin lymphoma or generalized Kaposi sarcoma); gastrointestinal manifestations such as chronic diarrhoea and dysphagia; neurological manifestations such as mono- and polyneuritis, AIDS dementia complex, (cryptococcal) meningitis and personality changes; pulmonary manifestations such as *M. tuberculosis* disease and *Streptococcus pneumoniae* or *Haemophilus influenzae* pneumonia; cardiac manifestations such as pericardial effusion (probably attributable to *M. tuberculosis* [212]); polylymphadenopathy; eye lesions which may be attributable to cytomegaly virus, toxoplasmosis or ophthalmic zoster; and haematological manifestations such as anaemia, leucopenia and lymphopenia.
    The clinical presentation of these diseases and their association with HIV-1 infection have been examined in a rather large number of hospital studies but in very few community-based studies [141]. Many of these hospital studies may have been adequate for describing the clinical presentation of diseases in HIV-1-infected individuals, but not for quantifying the association with HIV-1 infection because of a lack of controls for comparison of HIV-1 prevalence [213–216] or an inadequate selection of controls [217,218]. However, some hospital studies did include adequate control groups and confirmed the association of HIV-1 infection with, for instance, herpes zoster [57,159,219], oral thrush [57,159,220], chronic diarrhoea [57,159,221], *Cryptosporidium* in duodenal biopsies in patients with chronic diarrhoea [222], tuberculosis [57,223], weight loss [57,159], fever [57,159], pruritic papular eruption [159], polylymphadeno-pathy [159], pericardial effusion [212], pneumonia [224], pyomyositis [224], *Salmonella typhimurium* and *Streptococcus pneumoniae* bacteraemia [171]; and an absence of association of HIV-1 infection with faecal mycobacteria as a cause for diarrhoea [225,226]. In other studies HIV-1 prevalence was so high in cases of chronic diarrhoea [227], herpes zoster [228,229], tuberculous lymphadenitis [228] and pleural effusion [231] that an association with HIV-1 infection was beyond doubt.

Few studies have been carried out which determined the incidence of HIV-1 associated diseases and the population attributable risk of HIV-1 infection for those diseases (tuberculosis being a notable exception). A major difficulty in setting up such studies is that many diseases of interest may be rare in the study populations to be followed, and that there are so many diseases which are potentially important on which studies might be focused. As a first step to the development of prospective studies on specific diseases, a comparison was made between the incidence of various clinical and laboratory diagnoses HIV-1 infected and non-HIV-1 infected individuals in a cohort study among factory workers in Mwanza [44] (see Chapter 9).

The association between HIV-1 and tuberculosis has been well studied in Africa. A high HIV prevalence was found in various groups of tuberculosis patients [230–236], and a high prevalence of tuberculosis in AIDS patients who died [173]. A strong association was found between HIV-1 infection and tuberculosis disease in hospital-based [223] and community-based case-control studies [237,238] (see Chapter 5). In a cohort study among women of childbearing age the incidence of tuberculosis was greatly increased in HIV-1-infected women [239]. In a number of African countries, including Tanzania, an increased incidence of tuberculosis has been reported, which is attributed to HIV infection [232,233,238,240,241].

HIV-1-infected people have a particularly increased risk for extra-pulmonary tuberculosis [235,242]; if they have pulmonary tuberculosis, it is more likely to be sputum-smear negative than in non-HIV-1-infected individuals [235,243]. There is limited evidence that among sputum smear positive patients, HIV-1-infected individuals are less infectious than non-HIV-1-infected people [244]. Tuberculosis responds to anti-tuberculosis treatment nearly as well in HIV-seropositive as in HIV-seronegative individuals [242], provided rifampicin-containing regimens are used [232,245,246], although side-effects such as skin rashes and Stevens-Johnson syndrome are more frequent in HIV-1-infected people [232,242,243,247,248]. Recurrence of tuberculosis is more likely in HIV infected individuals, in particular when regimens do not include rifampicin [246,249], or when cutaneous hypersensitivity reactions necessitate substitution of thiacetazone by ethambutol [250]. In addition, mortality in HIV-1-infected tuberculosis patients is high [234,243,245,249], usually due to non-tuberculosis, HIV-related complications [242,245]. The effectiveness, feasibility and cost of targeted chemoprophylaxis is still a subject for further study [251,252].

On the association between HIV-1 infection and leprosy, much less is known. In a small, hospital-based, case-control study an association was shown between HIV-1 infection and newly diagnosed leprosy [253], but this was not confirmed in other hospital-based [254,255] or community-based [237] studies. The study presented in Chapter 6 [256] shows evidence of the association between HIV-1 and multibacillary leprosy from a community-based, case-control study and discusses possible reasons why this association has not been identified in some of the other studies. These include the long incubation period of leprosy [257] and of HIV infection, the relative rarity of leprosy, and the different distribution of HIV and leprosy: HIV is predominantly urban and leprosy predominantly rural [256]. Probably because not many HIV-1-infected leprosy patients have been seen yet, information on the clinical presentation and response to therapy of leprosy in HIV-1 infected people is still very limited [258].

Most studies have failed so far to demonstrate an association between HIV-1 infection and malaria, although the association was expected to be present because of the role of CD4 lymphocytes in immunity against malaria and the decline of CD4 in the course of HIV-1 infection [259–261]. In cross-sectional studies no association was found between asymptomatic malaria parasitaemia and HIV-1 infection [262], nor between clinical malaria and HIV-1 infection in hospital patients [263–266] or in those who died in hospital [173,267]. Prospective studies showed a few positive findings, including an increased incidence of fever with malaria parasitaemia in HIV-1 infected people [256], a non-significant relative risk for getting malaria of 1.6 in young children with AIDS [268], and an increased geometric mean parasite density in children with HIV-1 infection [269].

In the factory cohort study presented in Chapter 9, it is shown that HIV-1 infected adult men were 1.8 times more likely than those without HIV-1 infection to have had an episode of malaria disease [44]. Further studies on the association between malaria and HIV-1 infection are recommended which should include measurement of CD4 cells to assess the degree of immunodeficiency [44].

Studies on HIV associated morbidity may contribute to the appropriate treatment for HIV associated disease within the constraints posed by limited diagnostic facilities and funds for drugs, as has been shown in the case of tuberculosis [232,245,247,249]; they might also contribute to the prevention of such morbidity [248,249]. For diseases other than tuberculosis guidelines on their clinical management exist as well [270]. These guidelines should be adapted by national programmes in Africa for relevant diseases and available resources [270]. This adaptation would benefit from more information on the natural history of HIV infection (including a valid system for staging the course of infection), and an evaluation of the effectiveness and feasibility of these guidelines under field conditions for selected (common) conditions. Therefore, much work remains to be done.

This study

The research presented in this thesis was carried out as part of the Tanzania-Netherlands Research Project on AIDS and HIV Infection in Mwanza Region (TANERA). Some background information on the TANERA Project, Mwanza Region, and Tanzania is presented in Chapter 2.

Chapter 3 describes the prevalence of and risk factors for HIV-1 infection in Mwanza Region, as determined in a general population survey. In Chapters 4 to 6 the survey results are used for comparative studies: in Chapter 4 to validate information on HIV-1 prevalence from other sources, and in Chapters 5 and 6 in case-control studies to determine the risk of HIV-1 infection for developing tuberculosis or leprosy disease.

Chapter 7 describes the establishment of a cohort study among urban factory workers which aimed at determining the incidence of HIV-1 and other STDs, assessing changes in risk behaviour and HIV-1/STD incidence after the introduction of interventions and outlining the natural history of HIV-1 infection. Prevalence of and risk factors for HIV-1 infection at intake of the first 1000 workers are reported as well.

Chapter 8 describes the sexual risk behaviour at intake of the cohort and Chapter 9 the results in the first two years of follow up on HIV-1 incidence and HIV-1-associated mortality and morbidity. A general discussion is presented in Chapter 10.

References

1. Global Programme on AIDS. Global strategy for the prevention and control of AIDS: 1992 update. WHA45/29. Geneva: World Health Organization, 1992.
2. Nkowane BJ. Prevalence and incidence of HIV infection in Africa: a review of data published in 1990. AIDS 1991;5(Suppl 1):S7-S15.
3. De Cock KM, Brun-Vésinet F, Soro B. HIV-1 and HIV-2 infections and AIDS in West Africa. AIDS 1991;5(Suppl 1):S21-S28.
4. World Health Organization. Acquired immunodeficiency syndrome (AIDS) - Data as at June 1993. Wkly Epidemiol Rec 1993;68:193-194.
5. Department of Economic and Social Development, Statistical Division. 1991 Demographic yearbook. New York: United Nations, 1992.
6. Chin J, Mann J. Global surveillance and forecasting of AIDS. Bull Wrld Hlth Org 1989;67:1-7.
7. Chin J. Public health surveillance of AIDS and HIV infections. Bull Wrld Hlth Org 1990;68:529-536.
8. Chin J. The epidemiology and projected mortality of AIDS. In, Disease and mortality in sub-Saharan Africa. Feachem RG, Jamison DT (Eds). Oxford: Oxford University Press, 1991:203-213.
9. Perriens JH, Nyst M, Kapita BM, Liambi A, Stuyft P van der, Piot P. Evaluation of a hospital-based clinical surveillance system for AIDS in Kinshasa, Zaire. AIDS 1991(Suppl 1):S17-S20.
10. Berkley S, Okware S, Naamara W. Surveillance for AIDS in Uganda. AIDS 1989;3:79-85.
11. Colebunders RL, Weniger BG, Curran JW. Trends in human immunodeficiency virus infection. Eur J Clin Microbiol Infect Dis 1989;8:505-508.
12. World Health Organzation. Provisional clinical case definition for AIDS. Wkly Epidemiol Rec 1986;61:72-73.
13. De Cock KM, Selik RM, Soro B, Gayle H, Colebunders RL. AIDS surveillance in Africa: a reappraisal of case definitions. BMJ 1991;303:1185-88.
14. Gilks CF. What use is a clinical case definition for AIDS in Africa? BMJ 1991;303:1189-90.
15. Slutkin G, Chin J, Tarantola D, Mann J. Sentinel surveillance for HIV infection: a method to monitor HIV infection trends in population groups. WHO/GPA/DIR/88.8. Geneva: World Health Organization, 1988.
16. Dondero TJ, Curran JW. Serosurveillance of human immunodeficiency virus infection. Am J Public Health 1991;81:561-562.
17. Editorial. Anonymous HIV testing. Lancet 1990;335:575-576.
18. Gill ON, Adler MW, Day NE. Monitoring the prevalence of HIV. Foundations of a programme of unlinked anonymous testing in England and Wales. BMJ 1989;299:1295-1298.
19. Global Programme on AIDS. Unlinked anonymous screening for the public health surveilllance of HIV infections. Proposed international guidelines. GPA/SFI/89.3. Geneva: World Health Organization, 1989.
20. Hully HF, Bettinger CJ, Gallaher MM, Keller NM, Wilson J, Mertz GJ. Comparison of HIV-antibody prevalence in patients consenting to and declining HIV-antibody testing in an STD clinic. JAMA 1988;260:935-938.

21. Barbacci M, Repke JT, Chaisson RE. Routine prenatal screening for HIV infection. Lancet 1991;337:709-11.
22. Bindels PJE. Resultaten van de screening op HIV- antistoffen bij zwangere vrouwen, bezoeksters van infertiliteitspoliklinieken en abortusklinieken in de regio Amsterdam in 1990. Ned Tijdschr Geneesk 1991;135:2123-2128.
23. Hoff R, Berardi VP, Weiblen BJ, et al. Seroprevalence of human immunodeficiency virus among childbearing women. New Engl J Med 1988;318:525-530.
24. Ippolito G, Costa F, Stegagno M, Angeloni P, Angeloni U, Guzzanti E. Blind serosurvey of HIV antibodies in newborns in 92 Italian hospitals: a method for monitoring the infection rate in women at time of delivery. J Acq Imm Def Syndr 1991;4:402-407.
25. Novick LF, Berns D, Stricoff R, Stevens R, Pass K, Wethers J. HIV seroprevalence in newborns in New York State. JAMA 1989;261:1745-1750.
26. Peckham CS, Tedder RS, Briggs M, et al. Prevalence of maternal HIV infection based on unlinked anonymous testing of newborn babies. Lancet 1990;335:516-19.
27. Rosenberg PS, Levy ME, Brundage JF, et al. Population monitoring of an urban HIV/AIDS epidemic. JAMA 1992;268:495-503.
28. Kigadye RM, Klokke A, Nicoll A, et al. Sentinel surveillance for HIV-1 among pregnant women in a developing country: 3 years experience and comparison with a population survey. AIDS 1993;7:849-855.
29. Temmerman M, Mohamed Ali F, Ndinya-Achola J, Moses S, Plummer FA, Piot P. Rapid increase of both HIV-1 infection and syphilis among pregnant women in Nairobi, Kenya. AIDS 1992;6:1181-1185.
30. National AIDS Control Programme. HIV/AIDS/STD surveillance. Report No 7. Dar es Salaam: Ministry of Health, 1992.
31. Borgdorff M, Barongo L, Jaarsveld E van, et al. Sentinel surveillance for HIV-1 infection: How representative are blood donors; outpatients with fever, anaemia, or sexually transmitted diseases; and antenatal clinic attenders in Mwanza Region, Tanzania? AIDS 1993;7:567-572.
32. Killewo J, Nyamuryekung'e K, Sandstrom A, et al. Prevalence of HIV-1 infection in the Kagera Region of Tanzania: a population-based study. AIDS 1990;4:1081-1085.
33. Barongo LR, Borgdorff MW, Mosha FF, et al. The epidemiology of HIV-1 infection in urban areas, roadside settlements and rural villages in Mwanza Region, Tanzania. AIDS 1992;6:1521-1528.
34. Global Programme on AIDS. The HIV/AIDS pandemic: 1993 overview. WHO/GPA/CNP/EVA/93.1. Geneva: World Health Organization, 1993.
35. Quinn TC, Mann JM, Curran JW, Piot P. AIDS in Africa: an epidemiological paradigm. Science 1986;234:955-963.
36. Piot P, Laga M, Ryder R, et al. The global epidemiology of HIV infection: continuity, heterogeneity, and change. J Acq Imm Def Syndr 1990;3:403-412.
37. Dixon DO, Rida WN, Fast PE, Hoth DF. HIV vaccine trials: some design issues including sample size calculation. J Acquir Immune Defic Syndr 1993;6:485-496.
38. Ryder RW, Piot P. Epidemiology of HIV-1 infection in Africa. Bailliere's Clinical Tropical Medicine and Communicable Diseases 1988;3:13-29.
39. Killewo JZJ, Sandstrom A, Bredberg Raden U, Mhalu FS, Biberfeld G, Wall S. Incidence of HIV-1 infection among adults in the Kagera region of Tanzania. Int J Epidemiol 1993;22:528-536.
40. Wawer MJ, Sewankambo NK, Berkley S, et al. Incidence of HIV-1 infection in a rural region of Uganda. BMJ 1994;308:171-173.

41. Mulder DW, Nunn AJ, Wagner HU, Kamali A, Kengeya-Kayondo JF. HIV-1 incidence and HIV-1-associated mortality in a rural Ugandan population cohort. AIDS 1994;8:87-92.

42. Mann JM, Francis H, Quinn TC, et al. HIV seroincidence in a hospital worker population. Ann Soc Belg Med Trop 1986;66:245-250.

43. N'galy B, Ryder RW, Bila K, et al. Human immunodeficiency virus infection among employees in an African hospital. New Engl J Med 1988;319:1123-1127.

44. Borgdorff MW, Barongo LR, Klokke AH, et al. HIV-1 incidence and HIV-1 associated mortality and morbidity in a cohort of urban factory workers in northwest Tanzania. (Submitted for publication).

45. Andersson S, Nauclér A, Norrgren H, Dias F, Johansson I, Biberfeld G. HIV-1, HIV-2, HTLV and Treponema pallidum infections in a cohort of police officers in Guinea-Bissau. Abstract PO-C07-2739. Berlin, IXth International Conference on AIDS, June 1993:673.

46. Allen S, Serufilira A, Bogaerts J, et al. Confidential HIV testing and condom promotion in Africa. JAMA 1992;268:3338-3343.

47. Hira SK, Mangrola SG, Mwale C, et al. Apparent vertical transmission of human immunodeficiency virus type 1 by breastfeeding in Zambia. J Pediatr 1990;117:421-424.

48. Plummer FA, Simonsen JN, Cameron DW, et al. Cofactors in male-female sexual transmission of human immunodeficiency virus type 1. J Infect Dis 1991;163:233-239.

49. Laga M, Manoka A, Kivuvu M, et al. Non-ulcerative sexually transmitted diseases as risk factors for HIV-1 transmission in women: results from a cohort study. AIDS 1993;7:95-102.

50. Zekeng L, Feldblum PJ, Oliver RM, Kaptue L. Barrier contraceptive use and HIV infection among high-risk women in Cameroon. AIDS 1993;7:725-731.

51. Kreiss J, Ngugi E, Holmes K, et al. Efficacy of nonoxynol 9 contraceptive sponge use in preventing heterosexual acquisition of HIV in Nairobi prostitutes. JAMA 1992;268:477-482.

52. Jama Ahmed H, Omar K, Yusuf Adan S, Mohamed Guled A, Grillner L, Bygdeman S. Syphilis and human immunodeficiency virus seroconversion during a 6-month follow-up of female prostitutes in Mogadishu, Somalia. Int J STD AIDS 1991;2:119-123.

53. Cameron DW, Simonsen JN, D'Costa LJ, et al. Female to male transmission of human immunodeficiency virus type 1: risk factors for seroconversion in men. Lancet 1989;ii:403-407.

54. Allen S, Tice J, Perre P van de, et al. Effect of serotesting with counselling on condom use and seroconversion among HIV discordant couples in Africa. BMJ 1992;304:1605-1609.

55. Kamenga M, Ryder RW, Jingu M, et al. Evidence of marked sexual behaviour change associated with low HIV-1 seroconversion in 149 married couples with discordant HIV-1 serostatus: experience at an HIV counselling center in Zaire. AIDS 1991;5:61-67.

56. Mann JM, Quinn TC, Francis H, et al. Prevalence of HTLV-III/LAV in household contacts of patients with confirmed AIDS and controls in Kinshasa, Zaire. JAMA 1986;256:721-724.

57. Melbye M, Njelesani EK, Bayley A, et al. Evidence for heterosexual transmission and clinical manifestations of human immunodeficiency virus infection and related conditions in Lusaka, Zambia. Lancet 1986;ii:1113-1115.

58. N'galy B, Ryder RW. Epidemiology of HIV infection in Africa. J Acq Imm Def Syndr 1988;1:551-558.

59. Piot P, Colebunders R, Laga M, Ndinya-Achola JO, Groen G van der, Plummer FA. AIDS in Africa: a public health priority. J Virol Methods 1987;17:1-10.

60. Piot P, Mann M. Bidirectional heterosexual transmission of human immunodeficiency virus (HIV). Ann Inst Pasteur/Virol 1987;138:125-132.

61. Piot P, Kreiss JK, Ndinya-Achola JO, Ngugi EN, Simonsen JN, Cameron DW, Taelman H, Plummer FA. Heterosexual transmission of HIV. AIDS 1987;1:199-206.
62. Piot P, Plummer FA, Mhalu FS, Lamboray JL, Chin J, Mann JM. AIDS: an international perspective. Science 1988;239:573-579.
63. Piot P, Carael M. Epidemiological and sociological aspects of HIV-infection in developing countries. Br Med Bull 1988;44:68-88.
64. Berkley S. Parenteral transmission of HIV in Africa. AIDS 1991;5(Suppl 1):S87-S92.
65. Ryder RW, Temmerman M. The effect of HIV-1 infection during pregnancy and the perinatal period on maternal and child health in Africa. AIDS 1991;5(Suppl 1):S75-S85.
66. Bassett MT, Latif AS, Katzenstein DA, Emmanuel JC. Sexual behaviour and risk factors for HIV infection in a group of male factory workers who donated blood in Harare, Zimbabwe. J Acq Imm Def Syndr 1992;5:556-559.
67. Chiasson MA, Stoneburner RL, Hildebrandt DS, Ewing WE, Telzak EE, Jaffe HW. Heterosexual transmission of HIV-1 associated with the use of smokable freebase cocaine (crack). AIDS 1991;5:1121-1126.
68. Clumeck N, Perre P van de, Carael M, Rouvroy D, Nzaramba D. Heterosexual promiscuity among African patients with AIDS. New Engl J Med 1985;313:182.
69. Goodgame RW. AIDS in Uganda - clinical and social features. New Engl J Med 1990;323:383-389.
70. Johnson AM, Laga M. Heterosexual transmission of HIV. AIDS 1988;2(Suppl 1):S49-S56.
71. Nzila N, Laga M, Thiam MA, et al. HIV and other sexually transmitted diseases among female prostitutes in Kinshasa. AIDS 1991;5:715-721.
72. Perre P van de, Clumeck N, Carael M, et al. Female prostitutes: a risk group for infection with human T-cell lymphotropic virus type III. Lancet 1985;ii:524-526.
73. Perre P van de, Polain B le, Carael M, et al. HIV antibodies in a remote rural area in Rwanda, Central Africa: an analysis of potential risk factors for HIV seropositivity. AIDS 1987;1:213-215.
74. Serwadda D, Wawer MJ, Musgrave SD, Sewankambo NK, Kaplan JE, Gray RH. HIV risk factors in three geographic strata of rural Rakai District, Uganda. AIDS 1992;6:983-989.
75. Allen S, Lindan C, Serufiliria A, et al. Human immunodeficiency virus infection in urban Rwanda - demographic and behavioral coorelates in a representative sample of childbearing women. JAMA 1991;66:1657-1663.
76. Diallo MO, Ackah AN, Lafontaine MF, et al. HIV-1 and HIV-2 infections in men attending sexually transmitted disease clinics in Abidjan, Côte d'Ivoire. AIDS 1992;6:581-585.
77. Nopsekorn T, Mastro TD, Sangkharomya S. HIV-1 infction in young men in northern Thailand. AIDS 1993;7:1233-1239.
78. Simonsen JN, Cameron DW, Gakinya MN, et al. Human immunodeficiency virus infection among men with sexually transmitted diseases. New Engl J Med 1988;319:274-278.
79. Feldblum PJ, Fortney JA. Condoms, spermicides, and the transmission of human immunodeficiency virus: a review of the literature. Am J Public Health 1988;78:52-54.
80. Lamptey P, Goodridge GAW. Condom issues in AIDS prevention in Africa. AIDS 1991;5(Suppl 1):S183-S191.
81. Feldblum PJ. Results from prospective studies of HIV-discordant couples. AIDS 1991;5:1265-1266.
82. Fischl MA, Dickinson GM, Scott GB, Klimas N, Fletcher MA, Parks W. Evaluation of heterosexual partners, children, and household contacts of adults with AIDS. JAMA 1987;257:640-644.
83. Laurian Y, Peynet J, Verroust F. HIV infection in sexual partners of HIV-seropositive patients with hemophilia (letter). New Engl J Med 1989;320:183 (and erratum New Engl J Med 1989;321:268).

84. Lazzarin A, Saracco A, Musicco M, Nicolosi A, Italian study group on HIV heterosexual transmission. Man-to- woman sexual transmission of the human immunodeficiency virus. Arch Intern Med 1991;151:2411-2416.

85. Mann J, Quinn TC, Piot P, et al. Condom use and HIV infection among prostitutes in Zaire (letter). New Engl J Med 1987;316:345.

86. Ngugi EN, Plummer FA, Simonsen N, et al. Prevention of transmission of human immunodeficiency virus in Africa: effectiveness of condom promotion and health education among prostitutes. Lancet 1988;ii:887-890.

87. Saracco A, Musicco M, Nicolosi A, et al. Man-to-woman sexual transmission of HIV: longitudinal study of 343 steady partners of infected men. J Acq Imm Def Syndr 1993;6:497-502.

88. World Health Organization. Sexually transmitted diseases - condoms for prevention of sexually transmitted diseases. Wkly Epidem Rec 1988;63:169-172.

89. Padian NS, Shiboski SC, Jewell NP. The effect of the number of exposures on the risk of heterosexual HIV transmission. J Infect Dis 1990;161:883-887.

90. European study group. Risk factors for male to female transmission of HIV. Br Med J 1989;298:411-415.

91. Laga M, Taelman H, Van der Stuyft P, Bonneux L, Vercauteren G, Piot P. Advanced immunodeficiency as a risk factor for heterosexual transmission of HIV. AIDS 1989;3:361-366.

92. Seidlin M, Vogler M, Lee E, Lee YS, Dubin N. Heterosexual transmission of HIV in a cohort of couples in New York City. AIDS 1993;7:1247-1254.

93. European study group on heterosexual transmission of HIV. Comparison of female to male and male to female transmission of HIV in 563 stable couples. BMJ 1992;304;809-813.

94. Carswell JW, Lloyd G, Howells J. Prevalence of HIV-1 in east African lorry drivers. AIDS 1989;3:759-761.

95. Jessamine PG, Plummer FA, Ndinya-Achola JO, et al. Human immunodeficiency virus, genital ulcers and the male foreskin: synergism in HIV-1 transmission. Scand J Infect Dis 1990;69(Suppl):181-186.

96. Kreiss JK, Koech D, Plummer FA, et al. AIDS virus infection in Nairobi prostitutes. New Engl J Med 1986;314:414-418.

97. Simonsen JN, Plummer FA, Ngugi EN. HIV infection among lower socioeconomic strata prostitutes in Nairobi. AIDS 1990;4:139-144.

98. Laga M, Nzila N, Goeman J. The interrelationship of sexually transmitted diseases and HIV infection: implications for the control of both epidemics in Africa. AIDS 1991;5(Suppl 1):S55-S63.

99. Meulen J ter, Mgaya HN, Chang-Claude J, et al. Risk factors for HIV infection in gynaecological inpatients in Dar es Salaam, Tanzania, 1988-1990. East Afr Med J 1992;69:688-692.

100. Miotti PG, Dallabetta G, Ndovi E, Liomba G, Saah AJ, Chiphangwi J. HIV-1 and pregnant women: associated factors, prevalence, estimate of incidence and role in fetal wastage in central Africa. AIDS 1990;4:733-736.

101. Perre P van de, Carael M, Nzaramba D, Zissis G, Kayihigi J, Butzler JP. Risk factors for HIV seropositivity in selected urban-based Rwandese adults. AIDS 1987;1:207-211.

102. Piot P, Laga M. Genital ulcers, other sexually transmitted diseases, and the sexual transmission of HIV. BMJ 1989;298:623-624.

103. Ryder RW, Ndilu M, Hassig SE, et al. Heterosexual transmission of HIV-1 among employees and their spouses at two large businesses in Zaire. AIDS 1990;4:725-732.

104. Mertens TE, Hayes RJ, Smith PG. Epidemiological methods to study the interaction between HIV infection and other sexually transmitted diseases. AIDS 1990;4:57-65.

105. Greenblatt RM, Lukehart SA, Plummer FA, et al. Genital ulceration as a risk factor for human immunodeficiency virus infection. AIDS 1988;2:47-50.

106. Bongaarts J, Reining P, Way P, Conant F. The relationship between male circumcision and HIV infection in African populations. AIDS 1989;3:373-377.

107. Moses S, Bradley JE, Nagelkerke NJD, Ronald AR, Ndinya-Achola JO, Plummer FA. Geographical patterns of male circumcision practices in Africa: association with HIV seroprevalence. Int J Epidemiol 1990;19:693-697.

108. Caldwell JC, Caldwell P. The nature and limits of the sub-Saharan African AIDS epidemic: evidence from geographical and other patterns. Health Transition Working Paper No. 19. Canberra: Health Transition Centre, University of Australia, 1993.

109. Carael M, Perre PH van de, Lepage PH, et al. Human immunodeficiency virus transmission among heterosexual couples in Central Africa. AIDS 1988;2:201-205.

110. Barongo LR, Borgdorff MW, Newell JN, et al. Intake of a cohort study of urban factory workers in northwest Tanzania: risk factors for HIV-1 infection. Trop Geograph Med 1994; 46:157–162.

111. Borgdorff MW, Barongo LR, Newell JN, et al. Sexual partner change and condom use among urban factory workers in northwest Tanzania. Genitourin Med 1994 (In press).

112. Moss GB, Clemetson D, D'Costa L, et al. Association of cervical ectopy with heterosexual transmission of human immunodeficiency virus: results of a study of couples in Nairobi, Kenya. J Infect Dis 1991;164:588-591.

113. Bird KD. The use of spermicide containing nonoxynol-9 in the prevention of HIV infection. AIDS 1991;5:791-796.

114. Voeller B. Spermicides for controlling the spread of HIV (letter). AIDS 1992;6:341-342.

115. Niruthisard S, Roddy RE, Chutivongse S. Use of nonoxynol-9 and reduction in rate of gonococcal and chlamydial cervical infections. Lancet 1992;339:1371-1375.

116. Plummer FA, Fowke K, Nagelkerke NJD, et al. Evidence of resistance to HIV among continuously exposed prostitutes in Nairobi, Kenya. Abstract WS-A07-3. Berlin, IXth International Conference on AIDS, June 1993: 23.

117. Berkley S, Naamara W, Okware S, et al. AIDS and HIV infection in Uganda - are more women infected than men? AIDS 1990;4:1237-1242.

118. Rwandan HIV seroprevalence study group. Nationwide community-based serological survey of HIV-1 and other human retrovirus infections in a central African country. Lancet 1989;i:941-943.

119. Wawer MJ, Serwadda D, Musgrave SD, Konde-Lule JK, Musagara M, Sewankambo NK. Dynamics of spread of HIV-1 infection in a rural district of Uganda. BMJ 1991;303:1303-1306.

120. Mathiot CC, Lepage C, Chouaib E, Georges-Courbot M, Georges AJ. HIV seroprevalence and male to female ratio in central Africa. Lancet 1990;335:672.

121. Johnson AM, Petherick A, Davidson SJ, et al. Transmission of HIV to heterosexual partners of infected men and women. AIDS 1989;3:367-372.

122. Carael M, Cleland J, Adeokun L, Collaborating Investigators. Overview and selected findings of sexual behaviour surveys. AIDS 1991;5(Suppl 1):S65-S74.

123. Biggar RJ. The AIDS problem in Africa. Lancet 1986;i:79-83.

124. Kane F, Alary M, Ndoye I, et al. Temporary expatriation is related to HIV-1 infection in rural Senegal. AIDS 1993;7:1261-1265.

125. Laukamm-Josten U, Ocheng D, Mwizarubi BK, et al. HIV, hepatitis B and hepatitis C seroprevalence in truckstops and nearby communities in Tanzania. Abstract PO-C07-2737. Berlin, IXth International Conference on AIDS, June 1993:673.

126. Morse DL, Lessner L, Medvesky MG, Glebatis DM, Novick LF. IV. Geographic distribution of newborn HIV seroprevalence in relation to four sociodemographic variables. Am J Public Health 1991;81(Suppl):25-29.

127. St Louis ME, Conway GA, Hayman CR, Miller C, Petersen LR, Dondero TJ. Human immunodeficiency virus in disadvantaged adolescents. JAMA 1991;266:2387-2391.

128. Fife D, Mode C. AIDS incidence and income. J Acquir Immune Defic Syndr 1992;5:1105-1110.

129. Fife D, Mode C. AIDS prevalence by income group in Philadelphia. J Acquir Immune Defic Syndr 1992;5:1111-1115.

130. Nunn AJ, Kengeya-Kayondo JF, Malamba SS, Seeley JA, Mulder DW. Risk factors for HIV-1 infection in adults in a rural Ugandan community: a population study. AIDS 1994;8:81-86.

131. Malamba SS, Wagner HU, Maude G, et al. Risk factors for HIV-1 infection in adults in a rural Ugandan community: a case-control study. AIDS 1994;8:253-257.

132. Piot P, Kapita BM, Were JBO, Laga M, Colebunders RL. AIDS in Africa: the first decade and challenges for the 1990s. AIDS 1991;5 (Suppl 1):S1-S5.

133. Lamptey P, Piot P. The handbook for AIDS prevention in Africa. Durham: Family Health International, 1990.

134. Heymann DL, Edstrom K. Strategies for AIDS prevention and control in sub-Saharan Africa. AIDS 1991;5(Suppl 1):S197-S208.

135. Potts M, Anderson R, Boiley MC. Slowing the spread of human immunodeficiency virus in developing countries. Lancet 1991;338:608-613.

136. Plummer FA, Nagelkerke NJD, Moses S., Ndinya-Achola JO, Bwayo J, Ngugi E. The importance of core groups in the epidemiology and control of HIV-1 infection. AIDS 1991;5 (Suppl 1):S169-S176.

137. Lamptey P, Potts M. Targeting of prevention programs in Africa. In, The handbook for AIDS prevention in Africa. Eds Lamptey P, Piot P. Durham: Family Health International, 1990:144-180.

138. Zwi AB, Cabral AJR. Identifying "high risk situations" for preventing AIDS. BMJ 1991;303:1527-1529.

139. Piot P, Hira S. Control and prevention of sexually transmitted diseases. In, The handbook for AIDS prevention in Africa. Eds Lamptey P, Piot P. Durham: Family Health International, 1990:83-104.

140. WHO study group on management of sexually transmitted diseases patients. Management of patients with sexually transmitted diseases: report of a WHO study group. WHO Technical Report Series 810. Geneva: World Health Organization, 1991.

141. Colebunders RL, Latif AS. Natural history and clinical presentation of HIV-1 infection in adults. AIDS 1991;5(Suppl 1):S103-S112.

142. Bachetti P, Moss AR. Incubation period of AIDS in San Francisco. Nature 1989;338:251-253.

143. Biggar RJ and the International Registry of Seroconverters. AIDS incubation in 1891 seroconverters from different exposure groups. AIDS 1990;4:1059-1066.

144. Hendriks JCM, Medley GF, Griensven GJP van, Coutinho RA, Heisterkamp SH, Druten HAM van. The treament-free incubation period of AIDS in a cohort of homosexual men. AIDS 1993;7:231-239.

145. Medley GF, Anderson RM, Cox DR, Billard L. Incubation period of AIDS in patients infected via blood transfusion. Nature 1987;328:719-721.

146. Longini IM, Scott WC, Byers RH, et al. Statistical analysis of the stages of HIV infection using a Markov model. Stat Med 1989;8:831-843.

147. Moss AR Baccheti P. Natural history of HIV infection. AIDS 1989;3:55-61.

148. Rutherford GW, Lifson AR, Hessol NA, et al. Course of HIV-1 infection in a cohort of homosexual and bisexual men: an 11 year follow up study. Br Med J 1990;301:1183-1188.

149. Ward JW, Bush TJ, Perkins HA, et al. The natural history of transfusion-associated infection with human immunodeficiency virus. New Engl J Med 1989;321:947-952.

150. Mariotto AB, Mariotti S, Pezzotti P, Rezza G, Verdecchia A. Estimation of the acquired immune deficiency syndrome incubation period in intravenous drug users: a comparison with male homosexuals. Am J Epidemiol 1992;135:428-437.

151. Stoneburner RL, Des Jarlais DC, Benezra D, et al. A larger spectrum of severe HIV-1-related disease in intravenous drug users in New York City. Science 1988;242:916-919.

152. Selwyn PA. Injection drug use, mortality, and the AIDS epidemic. Am J Public Health 1991;81:1247-1249.

153. Selwyn PA, Alcabes P, Hartel D, et al. Clinical manifestations and predictors of disease progression in drug users with human immunodeficiency virus infection. N Engl J Med 1992;327:1697-1703.

154. Centers for Disease Control. 1993 revised classification system for HIV infection and expanded surveillance case definition for AIDS among adolescents and adults. MMWR 1992;41,No RR-17.

155. Brettle RP, Gore SM, Bird G, McNeil AJ. Clinical and epidemiological implications of the Centers for Disease Control/World Health Organization reclassification of AIDS cases. AIDS 1993;7:531-539.

156. Chaisson RE, Stanton DL, Gallant JE, Rucker S, Bartlett JG, Moore RD. Impact of the 1993 revision of the AIDS case definition on the prevalence of AIDS in a clinical setting. AIDS 1993;7:857-862.

157. Mientjes GHC, Ameijden EJC van, Keet RMP, Deutekom H van, Hoek JAR van den, Coutinho RA. Disproportional impact of the revised AIDS surveillance definition on the AIDS incidence among drug sers compared to homosexual men. (Submitted for publication).

158. Sabin C, Le CA, Phillips AN. New AIDS definition (letter). Lancet 1993;341:178.

159. Colebunders RL, Mann JM, Francis H, et al. Evaluation of a clinical case-definition of acquired immunodeficiency syndrome in Africa. Lancet 1987;i:492-494.

160. Widy-Wirski R, Berkley S, Downing R, et al. Evaluation of the WHO clinical case definition for AIDS in Uganda. JAMA 1988;260:3286-3289.

161. Wabwire-Mangen F, Serwadda D, Sewankambo NK, et al. Further experience with the World Health Organization clinical case definition for AIDS in Uganda (letter). AIDS 1989;3:462-463.

162. Lindan CP, Allen S, Serufilira A, et al. Predictors of mortality among HIV-infected women in Kigali, Rwanda. Ann Intern Med 1992;116:320-328.

163. Nagelkerke NJD, Plummer FA, Holton D, et al. Transition dynamics of HIV disease in a cohort of African prostitutes: a Markov model approach. AIDS 1990;4:743-747.

164. Bulterys M, Nzabihimana E, Chao A, et al. Long-term survival among HIV-1-infected prostitutes (letter). AIDS 1993;7:1269.

165. World Health Organization. Acquired immune deficiency syndrome (AIDS): interim proposal for a WHO staging system for HIV infection and disease. Wkly Epidemiol Rec 1990;65:221-228.

166. Montaner JSG, Le TN, Le N, Craib KJP, Schechter MT. Application of the World Health Organization system for HIV infection in a cohort of homosexual men in developing a prognostically meaningful staging system. AIDS 1992;6:719-724.

167. The WHO International Collaborating Group for the study of the WHO staging system. Proposed 'World Health Organization staging system for HIV infection and disease': preliminary testing by an international collaborative cross-sectional study. AIDS 1993;7:711-718.

168. Lima LAA, May SB, Perez MA, Schechter M. Survival of HIV-infected Brazilians: a model based on the World Health Organization staging system (letter). AIDS 1993;7:295-296.

169. De Cock KM et al. AIDS - the leading cause of death in the west African city of Abidjan, Ivory Coast. Science 1990;249:793-796.

170. De Cock KM, Porter A, Odehouri K, et al. Rapid emergence of AIDS in Abidjan, Ivory Coast. Lancet 1989;ii:408-411.

171. Gilks CF, Brindle RJ, Otieno LS, et al. Life-threatening bacteraemia in HIV-1 seropositive adults admitted to hospital in Nairobi, Kenya. Lancet 1990;336:545-549.

172. Hassig SE Perriens J, Baende E, et al. An analysis of the economic impact of HIV infection among patients at Mama Yemo Hospital, Kinshasa, Zaire. AIDS 1990;4:883-887.

173. Lucas SB, Hounnou A, Peacock C, et al. The mortality and pathology of HIV infection in a West African city. AIDS 1993;7:1569-1579.

174. Mbaga JM, Pallangyo KJ, Bakari M, Aris EA. Survival time of patients with acquired immune deficiency syndrome: experience with 274 patients in Dar-es-Salaam. East Afr Med J 1990;67:95-99.

175. Nelson AM et al, Hassig SE, Kayembe M, et al. HIV-1 seropositivity and mortality at University Hospital, Kinshasa, Zaire,1987. AIDS 1991;5:583-586.

176. Muller O, Moser R. HIV-1 disease in a Kampala hospital 1985-89 (letter). Lancet 1990;335:236-237.

177. Ryder RW, Batter VL, Nsuami M, et al. Fertility rates in 238 HIV-1-seropositive women in Zaire followed for 3 years post-partum. AIDS 1991;5:1521-1527.

178. Konde-Lule JK, Zirabamuzale C. The long term impact data is beginning to come in: results of a 30 month population-based HIV study in peri urban Uganda. Abstract MC 3211. Florence, VIIth International Conference on AIDS, June 1991:350.

179. Anderson RM, May RM, Boily MC, Garnett GP, Rowley JT. The spread of HIV-1 in Africa: sexual contact patterns and the predicted demographic impact of AIDS. Nature 1991;352:581-589.

180. Anderson RM. Some aspects of sexual behaviour and the potential demographic impact of AIDS in developing countries. Soc Sci Med 1992;34:271-280.

181. Anderson RM. AIDS and its demographic impact. In, Disease and mortality in sub-Saharan Africa. Feachem RG, Jamison DT (Eds). Oxford: Oxford University Press, 1991:203-213.

182. Mientjes G. Studies on the natural course of HIV infection among injecting drug users. Amsterdam: Academisch Proefschrift, Universiteit van Amsterdam, 1993:86-104.

183. Blaxhult A, Granath F, Lidman K, Giesecke J. The influence of age on the latency period to AIDS in people infected by HIV through blood transfusion. AIDS 1990;4:125-129.

184. Gardner LI, Brundage JF, McNeil JG, et al. Predictors of HIV-1 disease progression in early- and late-stage patients: the U.S. army natural history cohort. J Acquir Immune Defic Syndr 1992;5:782-793.

185. Lange JMA, Wolf F de, Goudsmit J. Markers for progression in HIV infection. AIDS 1989;3(Suppl 1):S153-S160.

186. Wenger JD, Whalen CC, Lederman MM, et al. Prognostic factors in acquired immunodeficiency syndrome. J Gen Intern Med 1988;3:464-470.

187. Phair J, Jacobson L, Detels R, et al. Acquired immune deficiency syndrome occurring within 5 years of infection with human immunodeficiency virus type-1: the Multicenter AIDS Cohort Study. J Acquir Immune Defic Syndr 1992;5:490-496.

188. Schechter MT, Craib KJP, Le TN, et al. Progression to AIDS and predictors of AIDS in seroprevalent and seroincident cohorts of homosexual men. AIDS 1989;3:347-353.

189. Griensven GJP van, Vroome EMM de, Wolf F de, Goudsmit J, Roos M, Coutinho RA. Risk factors for progression of human immunodeficiency virus (HIV) infection among seroconverted and seropositive homosexual men. Am J Epidemiol 1990;132:203-210.

190. Keet IPM, Krijnen P, Koot M, et al. Predictors of rapid progression to AIDS in HIV-1 seroconverters. AIDS 1993;7:51-57.

191. Munoz A, Vlahov D, Solomon L, et al. Prognostic indicators for development of AIDS among intravenous drug users. J Acquir Immune Defic Syndr 1992;5:694-700.
192. Phillips AN, Lee CA, Elford J. Serial CD4 lymphocyte counts and development of AIDS. Lancet 1991;337:389-392.
193. Chlebowski RT, Grosvenor MB, Bernhard NH, Morales NS, Bulcavage LM. Nutritional status, gastrointestinal dysfunction, and survival in patients with AIDS. Am J Gastroenterol 1989;84:1288-1293.
194. Murray HW, Godbold JH, Jurica KB, Roberts RB. Progression to AIDS in patients with lymphadenopathy or AIDS-related complex: reappraisal of risk and predictive factors. Am J Med 1989;86:533-538.
195. Kramer A, Biggar RJ, Hampl H, et al. Immunologic markers of progression to acquired immune deficiency syndrome are time-dependent and illness-specific. Am J Epidemiol 1992;136:71-80.
196. Moss AR, Bacchetti P, Osmond D, et al. Seropositivity for HIV and the development of AIDS or AIDS related condition: three year follow up of the San Francisco General Hospital cohort. Br Med J 1988;296:745-750.
197. Lifson AR, Hessol NA, Buchbinder SP, et al. Serum β_2-microglobulin and prediction of progression to AIDS in HIV infection. Lancet 1992;339:1436-1440.
198. Saah AJ, Munoz A, Kuo V, et al. Predictors of the risk of development of acquired immune deficiency syndrome within 24 months among gay men seropositive for human immunodeficiency virus type 1: a report from the Multicentre AIDS Cohort Study. Am J Epidemiol 1992;135:1147-1155.
199. Dax EM. HIV testing and staging, disease progression, and markers. Current Opinion in Infectious Diseases 1993;6:191-199.
200. Schellekens PTA, Tersmette M, Roos MTL, et al. Biphasic rate of CD4+ cell count decline during progression to AIDS correlates with HIV-1 phenotype. AIDS 1992;6:665-669.
201. Moss AR. Predicting who will progress to AIDS. BMJ 1988;297:1067-1068.
202. Simmonds P, Beatson D, Cuthbert RJG, et al. Determinants of HIV disease progression: six-year longitudinal study in the Edinburgh haemophilia/HIV cohort. Lancet 1991;338:1159-1163.
203. Tersmette M, Lange JMA, De Goede REY, et al. Differences in risk for AIDS and AIDS mortality associated with biological properties of HIV variants. Lancet 1989;i:983-985.
204. Koot M, Vos AHV, Keet RPM, et al. HIV-1 biological phenotype in long-term infected individuals evaluated with an MT-2 cocultivation assay. AIDS 1992;6:49-54.
205. Tersmette M, Schuitemaker H. Virulent HIV strains? AIDS 1993;7:1123-1125.
206. Steel CM Ludlam CA, Beatson D, et al. HLA haplotype A1 B8 DR3 as a risk factor for HIV-related disease. Lancet 1990;i:1185-1188.
207. Kaslow RA, Duquesnoy R, Van Raden M, et al. A1 Cw7 B8 DR3 HLA antigen combination associated with rapid decline of T-helper lymphocytes in HIV-1 infection. Lancet 1990;335:927-930.
208. Baillou A, Barin F, Allain J, et al. Human immunodeficiency virus antigenemia in patients with AIDS and AIDS-related disorders: a comparison between European and Central African populations. J Infect Dis 1987;156:830-833.
209. Jorgensen AF, Jensen VG, Shao JF, et al. Beta$_2$-microglobulin as a prognostic marker for patients with AIDS in Dar es Salaam, Tanzania (letter). AIDS 1990;4:1168-1169.
210. Whittle H, Eboga A, Todd J, et al. Clinical and laboratory predictors of survival in Gambian patients with symptomatic HIV-1 or HIV-2 infection. AIDS 1992;6:685-689.
211. Gonzales-Clemente JM, Miro JM, Navarro MP, Zamora L, Vilardell E. High triglyceride levels as a predictor for mortality in AIDS patients (letter). AIDS 1993;7:1022-1023.

212. Cegielski JP, Ramaiya K, Lallinger GJ, Mtulia IA, Mbaga IM. Pericardial disease and human immunodeficiency virus in Dar es Salaam, Tanzania. Lancet 1990;335:209-212.

213. Gilks CF, Ojoo SA, Brindle RJ. Non-opportunistic bacterial infections in HIV-seropositive adults in Nairobi, Kenya. AIDS 1991;5(Suppl 1):S113-S116.

214. Hira SK, Wadhawan D, Kamanga J, et al. Cutaneous manifestations of human immunodeficiency virus in Lusaka, Zambia. J Am Acad Dermatol 1988;19:451-457.

215. McLeod DT, Neill P, Gwanzura L, et al. Pneumocystis carinii pneumonia in patients with AIDS in Central Africa. Resp Med 1990;84:225-228.

216. McLeod DT, Neill P, Robertson VJ, et al. Pulmonary diseases in patients infected with the human immunodeficiency virus in Zimbabwe, Central Africa. Trans Roy Soc Trop Med Hyg 1989;83:694-697.

217. Howlett WP, Nkya WM, Mmumi KA, Missalek WR. Neurological disorders in AIDS and HIV disease in the northern zone of Tanzania. AIDS 1989;3:289-296.

218. Belec L, Di Constanzo B, Georges AJ, Gherardi R. HIV infection in African patients with pyomyositis (letter). AIDS 1991;5:234.

219. Colebunders R, Mann JM, Francis H, et al. Herpes zoster in African patients: a clinical predictor of human immunodeficiency virus infection. J Infect Dis 1988;157:314-318.

220. Magaruka Z, Perriens JH, Kapita B, Piot P. Oral manifestations of HIV-1 infection in Zairian patients (letter). AIDS 1991;5:237-238.

221. Conlon CP, Pinching AJ, Perera CU, Moody A, Luo NP, Lucas SB. HIV-related enteropathy in Zambia: a clinical, microbiological and histological study. Am J Trop Med Hyg 1990;42:83-88.

222. Colebunders R, Lusakumuni K, Nelson AM, et al. Persistent diarrhoea in Zairian AIDS patients: an endoscopic and histological study. Gut 1988;29:1687-1691.

223. De Cock KM, Gnaore E, Adjorlolo G, et al. Risk of tuberculosis in patients with HIV-I and HIV-II infections in Abidjan, Ivory Coast. BMJ 191;302:496-499.

224. Pallangyo K, Hakanson A, Lema L, et al. High HIV seroprevalence and increased HIV-associated mortality among hospitalized patients with deep bacterial infections in Dar es Salaam, Tanzania. AIDS 1992;6:971-976.

225. Conlon CP, Banda HM, Luo NP, Namaambo MKM, Perera CU, Sikweze J. Faecal mycobacteria and their relationship to HIV-related enteritis in Lusaka, Zambia. AIDS 1989;3:539-541.

226. Colebunders R, Nembunzu M, Portaels F, Lusakumumu K, Kapita B, Piot P. Isolation of mycobacteria from stools and intestinal biopsies from HIV seropositive and HIV seronegative patients with and without diarrhea in Kinshasa, Zaire. Ann Soc Belg Med Trop 1990;70:303-309.

227. Colebunders R, Francis H, Mann JM, et al. Persistent diarrhea strongly associated with HIV infection in Kinshasa, Zaire. Am J Gastroenterol 1987;82:859-864.

228. Perre P van de, Bakkers E, Batungwanayo J, et al. Herpes zoster in African patients: an early manifestation of HIV infection. Scand J Infect Dis 1988;20:277-282.

229. Dehne KL, Dhlakama DG, Richter C, Mawadza M, McClean D, Huss R. Herpes zoster as an indicator of HIV infection in Africa. Trop Doctor 1992;22:68-70.

230. 228.Nambuya A, Sewankambo N, Mugerwa J, Goodgame R, Lucas S. Tuberculous lymphadenitis associated with human immunodeficiency virus (HIV) in Uganda. J Clin Pathol 1988;41:93-96.

231. Batungwanayo J, Taelman H, Allen S, Bogaerts J, Kagame A, Perre P van de. Pleural effusion, tuberculosis and HIV-1 infection in Kigali, Rwanda. AIDS 1993;7:73-79.

232. De Cock KM, Soro B, Coulibaly IM, Lucas SB. Tuberculosis and HIV infection in sub-Saharan Africa. JAMA;268:1581-1587.

233. Harries AD. Tuberculosis and human immunodeficiency virus infection in developing countries. Lancet 1990;335:387-390.

234. Colebunders RL, Ryder RW, Nzilambi N, et al. HIV infection in patients with tuberculosis in Kinshasa, Zaire. Am Rev Respir Dis 1989;139:1082-1085.

235. Elliott AM, Luo N, Tembo G, et al. Impact of HIV on tuberculosis in Zambia: a cross sectional study. Br Med J 1990;301:412-415.

236. Kelly P, Burnham G, Radford C. HIV seropositivity and tuberculosis in a rural Malawi hospital. Trans Roy Soc Trop Med Hyg 1990;84:725-727.

237. Pönnighaus JM, Mwanjasi LJ, Fine PEM, et al. Is HIV infection a risk factor for leprosy? Int J Lepr 1991;59:221-228.

238. Broek J van den, Borgdorff MW, Pakker NG, et al. HIV-1 infection as a risk factor for the development of tuberculosis disease: a population-based case-control study in Tanzania. Int J Epidemiol 1993;22:1159-1165.

239. Braun MM, Badi N, Ryder RW, et al. A retrospective cohort study of the risk of tuberculosis among women of childbearing age with HIV infection in Zaire. Am Rev Respir Dis 1991;143:501-504.

240. Murray JF. Tuberculosis and human immunodeficiency virus infection during the 1990's. Bull Int Union Tuberc Lung Dis 1991;66:21-25.

241. Broekmans JP. Tuberculosis and HIV-infection in developing countries. Trop Geograph Med 1991;43(Suppl):S13-S21.

242. Perriens JH, Mukadi Y, Nunn P. Tuberculosis and HIV infection: implications for Africa. AIDS 1991;5:(Suppl 1):S127-S133.

243. Kochi A. Government intervention programs in HIV/tuberculous infection. Bull Int Union Tuberc Lung Dis 1991;66:33-36.

244. Elliott AM, Hayes RJ, Halwindii B, et al. The impact of HIV on infectiousness of pulmonary tuberculosis: a community study in Zambia. AIDS 1993;7:981-987.

245. Nunn P, Brindle R, Carpenter L, et al. Cohort study of human immunodeficiency virus infection in patients with tuberculosis in Nairobi, Kenya. Am Rev Respir Dis 1992;146:849-854.

246. Daley G. Tuberculosis recurrence in Africa: true relapse or re-infection? Lancet 1993;342:756-757.

247. Nunn P Kibuga D, Gathua S, et al. Cutaneous hypersensitivity reactions due to thiacetazone in HIV-1 seropositive patients treated for tuberculosis. Lancet 1991;337:627-630.

248. World Health Organization. Severe hypersensitivity reactions among HIV-seropositve patients with tuberculosis treated with thioacetazone. Wkly Epidemiol Rec 1992;67:1-3.

249. Perriens JH, Colebunders RL, Karakunga C, et al. Increased mortality and tuberculosis treatment failure rate among human immunodeficiency virus (HIV) seropositive compared with HIV seronegative patients with pulmonary tuberculosis treated with "standard" chemotherapy in Kinshasa, Zaire. Am Rev Respir Dis 1991;144:750-755.

250. Hawken M, Nunn P, Gathua S, et al. Increased recurrence of tuberculosis in HIV-1 infected patients in Kenya. Lancet 1993;342:332-337.

251. Narain JP, Slutkin G, Dam HG ten, Kochi A. Preventive tuberculosis chemotherapy in HIV infection: a priority for study (letter). AIDS 1992;6:744-746.

252. Nairain JP, Raviglione MC, Kochi A. HIV-associated tuberculosis in developing countries: epidemiology and strategies for prevention. WHO/TB/92.166. Geneva: World Health Organization, 1992.

253. Meeran K. Prevalence of HIV infection among patients with leprosy and tuberculosis in rural Zambia. Br Med J 1989;298:364-365.

254. Tekle-Haimanot R, Frommel D, Tadesse T, Verdier M, Abebe M, Denis F. A survey of HTLV-1 and HIVs in Ethiopian leprosy patients (letter). AIDS 1991;5:108-110.

255. Leonard G, Sangare A, Verdier M, et al. Prevalence of HIV infection among patients with leprosy in African countries and Yemen. J Acq Imm Def Syndr 1990;3:1109-1113.

256. Borgdorff MW, Broek J van den, Chum H, et al. HIV-1 infection as a risk factor for leprosy: a case-control study in Tanzania. Int J Leprosy 1993;61:556-562.

257. Turk JL, Rees RJW. AIDS and leprosy. Lepr Rev 1988;59:193-194.

258. Vreeburg AEM. Clinical observations on leprosy patients with HIV1-infection in Zambia. Lepr Rev 1992;63:134-140.

259. Colebunders R, Bahwe Y, Nekwei W, et al. Incidence of malaria and efficacy of oral quinine in patients recently infected with human immunodeficiency virus in Kinshasa, Zaire. J Infection 1990;21:167-173.

260. Lucas SB. Missing infections in AIDS. Trans Roy Soc Trop Med Hyg 1990;84(Suppl 1):34-38.

261. Butcher GA. HIV and malaria: a lesson in immunology? Parasitology Today 1992;8:307-311.

262. Allen S, Van de perre P, Serufilira A, et al. Human immunodeficiency virus and malaria in a representative sample of childbearing women in Kigali, Rwanda. J Infect Dis 1991;164:67-71.

263. Muller O, Musoke P, Sen G, Moser R. Pediatric HIV-1 disease in a Kampala hospital. J Trop Pediatr 1990;36:283-286.

264. Muller O, Moser R. The clinical and parasitological presentation of Plasmodium falciparum malaria is unaffected by HIV-1 infection. Trans Roy Soc trop Med Hyg 1990;84:336-338.

265. Simooya OO, Mwendapole RM, Siziya S, Fleming AF. Relation between falciparum malaria and HIV seropositivity in Ndola, Zambia. Br Med J 1988;297:30-31.

266. Simooya OO, Mwendapole RM, Sikateyo BM. Severe falciparum malaria and the acquired immunodeficiency syndrome (AIDS) in Zambia (letter). Ann Trop Med Parasitol 1991;85:269-270.

267. Muller O, Moser R, Guggenberger P, Alexander M. AIDS in Africa (letter). New Engl J Med 1991;324:847-848

268. Greenberg AE, Nsa W, Ryder RW, et al. Plasmodium falciparum malaria and perinatally acquired human immunodeficiency virus type 1 infection in Kinshasa, Zaire. New Engl J Med 1991;325:105-109.

269. Shaffer N, Hedberg K, Davachi F, et al. Trends and risk factors for HIV-1 seropositivity among outpatient children, Kinshasa, Zaire. AIDS 1990;4:1231-1236.

270. Global Programme on AIDS. Guidelines for the clinical management of HIV infection in adults. Geneva: World Health Organization, 1991.

2

Tanzania-Netherlands Research Project on AIDS and HIV Infection in Mwanza Region (TANERA)

In this chapter some background information is presented on Tanzania and Mwanza Region and on the Tanzania-Netherlands Research Project on AIDS and HIV Infection in Mwanza Region (TANERA).

Mwanza Region, Tanzania

The United Republic of Tanzania is situated in East Africa just below the Equator (see Figure 1 in Chapter 1). Its neighbouring countries are (anti-clockwise starting north) Kenya, Uganda, Rwanda, Burundi, Zaire, Zambia, Malawi, and Mozambique. The country covers an area of 945,000 km^2 [1] and had in 1991 a population of 28 million [2]. Of the total population 79% lived in rural areas in 1990. Some other demographic, as well as social and economic statistics of Tanzania are presented in Table 1. For comparison, data of the Netherlands are given as well.

Tanzania mainland (Tanganyika) was a German colony from 1890 to 1919 [1], and a British Mandate from the League of Nations from 1919 to 1961. In 1961 it became independent; in 1964 it joined with Zanzibar to form the United Republic of Tanzania. The official language is Swahili.

Tanzania belongs to the low income countries with a gross national product (GNP) per capita of $100 in 1991 [3]. Agriculture comprised 61% of the gross domestic product in 1990, services 34% and industry 5%. Foreign debt in 1991 was $ 6,460 million, i.e. 2.5 times the GNP [3]. Government policy was socialist oriented under President Nyerere (1961–1985), but has been shifting gradually towards a free market orientation under President Mwinyi since 1985 [1].

As the crude birth rate in Tanzania is high at 48/1000, a high proportion (48%) of people are less than 15 years old, and the annual population growth is also high at 3.3% [4]. Life expectancy at birth is 53 years. This is influenced to a large extent by the high infant mortality rate (112/1000 in 1991) and under-five mortality rate (178/1000 in 1991) [5]. Major causes of death in Tanzania are malnutrition and infectious diseases such as malaria, acute respiratory infections, diarrhoeal diseases, tuberculosis and AIDS, and problems related to pregnancy and childbirth [6,7], as is the case in other developing countries [8–10].

Tanzania has adopted a primary health care policy, which aims at improving health

Table 1. **Some demographic, social, and economic statistics of Tanzania and the Netherlands**

		Tanzania	Netherlands
Size (km^2)		945 087	40 844
Population (1990)		25.6 million	14.9 million
Population density		30/km^2	369/km2
Urban population (1990)		21%	89%
Annual population growth		3.3%	0.6%
Crude birth rate (1991)		48/1000	13/1000
Crude death rate (1991)		15/1000	9/1000
Pop. aged <15 year		48%	18%
Infant mortality rate (1991)		112/1000	7/1000
Under-five mortality rate (1991)		178/1000	8/1000
Life expectancy (1990)	M	50 year	74 year
	F	54 year	80 year
Adult literacy rate (1990)	M	93%	99%
	F	88%	99%
School enrolment ratio primary school (1986-90)	M	47	100
	F	48	100
School enrolment ratio secondary school (1986-90)	M	5	105
	F	4	102
GNP per capita (1990)		$ 120	$ 17 320
Annual GNP per capita growth rate (1980-90)		-0.7%	1.4%
ODA as % of GNP		42%	n/a

Sources: references 1, 2, 3, 4 and 5

for all inhabitants through health services, community participation, and intersectoral collaboration. Elements include an integrated maternal and child health programme, expanded programme on immunization, essential drugs programme, control of diarrhoeal disease through promotion of oral rehydration therapy, and programmes to train village health workers and traditional birth attendants [11,12].

The health care system is hierarchical and links up with a subdivision of the country according to levels of local government [11,12]. Supervisors of curative and preventive health services at regional and district levels are situated in the regional and district medical offices, respectively, which are part of the local government structure. Levels of care include zonal and regional referral hospitals (highest cadre: specialists), district hospitals (medical officers), health centres (medical assistants), dispensaries (rural medical aides), and village health posts (village health workers and traditional birth attendants). Churches are an important provider of health services at all levels. An expansion of government health services combined with a reduction in per capita expenditure on health by the government has led to problems with the quality of services [1,7,11,12].

Mwanza Region is situated in the northwest of Tanzania along the shores of Lake Victoria. It covers a land area of 19,500 km^2 and had in 1990 a population of 1,981,000 (based on an extrapolation of the 1978 and 1988 census results); the intercensus growth rate was 2.7% [13]. In Tanzania it is the Region with the largest population and the greatest population density after Dar es Salaam.

Main sources of income are agriculture (e.g. cotton, rice, maize, cassava), fishing (Lake Victoria), services (e.g. banks, transport), and a limited industrial production (e.g. textile, soft drinks). Mwanza functions as a trade centre in northwest Tanzania, as it is situated at Lake Victoria (trade with Uganda) and along main roads to Kenya, Rwanda, Burundi, and Dar es Salaam.

The largest tribes in the region are Sukuma, Zinza, and Kerewe, although much mixing with other tribes occurs, particularly in town. The major religious denominations are Roman Catholic, African Inland Church, a variety of other protestant churches, and Islam.

TANERA Project

After the first cases of AIDS had been notified in Tanzania in 1983 [14], the size of the AIDS/HIV problem increased rapidly. The Ministry of Health established a National AIDS Task Force in 1985, formulated a first medium term plan on AIDS control for 1987–1992, and established a National AIDS Control Programme (NACP) in 1988. A second medium term plan has been formulated for the period 1992–1996. It aims at reducing HIV transmission and at alleviating the personal and social impact of HIV infection and AIDS [15]. Compared with the first medium term plan, much more emphasis is put on decentralisation to district level and on multisectoral collaboration in AIDS control.

Because of the large perceived threat of the AIDS epidemic, the Government of Tanzania has sought donor support for AIDS control from various countries. In 1987 the Netherlands Minister for Development Cooperation sent a mission to Mwanza Region in order to identify what support the Netherlands might give towards AIDS control in this region [16,17,18]. This led to the establishment of two projects, both funded by the Netherlands Minister for Development Cooperation. The first one to start was named 'Prevention of AIDS and Hepatitis B in Tanzania' and took place from 1989 to 1990. It was a collaborative project between Bugando Medical Centre and the Nijmegen Institute for International Health and aimed at the introduction of HIV test kits in the region in order to reduce HIV transmission by blood transfusion [19,20].

The second project was the Tanzania-Netherlands Research Project on AIDS and HIV

Infection in Mwanza Region (TANERA), which started in 1990. Its birth was rather complicated. Bugando Medical Centre and the Nijmegen Institute for International Health had planned (as a continuation of the 'Prevention of AIDS and Hepatitis B in Tanzania' project) further studies on medical care-related transmission and a population survey. At the same time, the National Institute for Medical Research and the Royal Tropical Institute had prepared a proposal for Multidisciplinary Research to Develop AIDS Control Methods (MURDAC), which comprised plans for epidemiological studies (population survey and factory cohort study) and social-behavioural studies (focusing on knowledge, attitudes, beliefs, and practices regarding sexual HIV transmission and on coping with AIDS by families and communities). At the request of the funding agency, these two proposals were merged into one, and the interests and priorities of various Tanzanian institutions (including Ministry of Health/NACP, Regional Medical Office Mwanza, and researchers from Muhimbili Medical Centre) were made explicit once more in a workshop in Dar es Salaam in August 1989.

As all parties agreed on what needed to be done, a formulation workshop took place in Mwanza in October/November 1989, in which research proposals were written up in more detail and agreement was reached about the administrative structure of the project and on issues such as authorship of scientific papers. These proposals were cleared by the Tanzanian Ministry of Health and accepted for funding by the Netherlands Minister for Development Cooperation in time for the project to start in April 1990. The decision to fund the project was provisional: funding was guaranteed for a first period of one year, funding for a second period of two years was dependent on the outcome of an evaluation which took place 10 months after the inception of the project.

The TANERA project aimed at contributing to the development of appropriate and effective methods for the reduction of HIV transmission. This was done through epidemiological, social-behavioural, and clinical studies, carried out under the responsibility of the Mwanza Medical Research Centre, Regional Medical Office, and Bugando Medical Centre, respectively. The TANERA Information, Education, and Communication (IEC) unit at the Regional Medical Office worked in close collaboration with the researchers on the development and implementation of interventions.

The epidemiological studies included a survey on the prevalence of sexually transmitted diseases (STD), including HIV infection, in Mwanza Region [21–23]; validation of sentinel surveillance [24,25]; and a cohort study among factory workers [26–28]. The prevalence survey and validation of sentinel surveillance were carried out in collaboration with the African Medical and Research Foundation (AMREF); the factory cohort study is still ongoing. Case-control studies on HIV-1 as a risk factor for tuberculosis and leprosy, which were carried out in collaboration with the National Tuberculosis and Leprosy Programme, were not planned originally, but were found to be possible with little extra effort while the project was in progress [29,30]. A study on risk factors for HIV-1 infection in rural areas was cancelled after it was clear that further cross-sectional studies were unlikely to provide new information, while setting up a prospective rural study was not feasible at that stage.

The social-behavioural research included a study on the knowledge, attitudes, beliefs and practices regarding AIDS, AIDS control measures, treatment seeking behaviour, and sexual relations and practices; a follow up study of AIDS patients and their families (relatives, households) in rural and urban areas; and a study to formulate, organize and evaluate selected AIDS control interventions in an area of Mwanza town [31].

The clinical studies were all intervention studies aiming at the reduction of medical care related transmission through blood transfusions [32–34] and injections [35,36], and the risk of occupational HIV transmission to health care workers. The studies on blood transfusions and injections were completed; the health worker study is ongoing.

The IEC Unit carried out a number of interventions among groups of barmaids, factory workers, and schoolchildren, including promotion of condoms, IEC on limiting the number of partners and promotion of early STD treatment. For barworkers this included a mobile STD clinic. Other interventions to which the project contributed were provision of medical care and counselling at the factory clinic; provision of tests for screening blood donors in Mwanza Region; and training health workers to reduce the number of avoidable blood transfusions and number of injections and to increase the use of sterile needles and syringes.

The project involved researchers from the disciplines of epidemiology, statistics, biochemistry, microbiology, clinical medicine, medical anthropology, and medical sociology. There was a close interdisciplinary collaboration within two clusters: epidemiology, statistics, microbiology, biochemistry, and clinical medicine on the one hand, and medical sociology and medical anthropology on the other. Between the two clusters collaboration took place on the implementation of interventions, though research collaboration was limited.

The project was conceived as a collaborative effort of three Tanzanian and two Dutch institutions: the Regional Medical Office of Mwanza, Mwanza Medical Research Centre, and Bugando Medical Centre in Tanzania and Royal Tropical Institute, Amsterdam and Nijmegen Institute for International Health in the Netherlands. The three Tanzanian institutions were responsible for the day-to-day implementation of the studies and interventions. The two Dutch institutions provided scientific and administrative support. The project had an extremely fruitful collaboration with AMREF's STD/HIV intervention project (which was supported by the London School of Hygiene and Tropical Medicine) and the National and Regional TB/Leprosy control programme.

Financial support to the project was given by the Netherlands Minister for Development Cooperation, through the Royal Tropical Institute. The Regional Medical Officer was the TANERA Project Coordinator. S/he was administratively supported by the Netherlands Project Leader. The author of this thesis was the Project Leader of the TANERA Project from April 1990 to September 1993 and shared in the same period responsibility for the epidemiological studies with his NIMR counterpart.

The TANERA Project completed its first main phase in December 1993. It is now continuing under the name TANESA: Tanzania-Netherlands Project to Support AIDS Control in Mwanza Region, Tanzania. In this project a number of research activities are continuing, but more emphasis is put on the support of a pilot district AIDS control programme.

References

1. Kussendrager N. Tanzania. Landenreeks. Amsterdam: Koninklijk Instituut voor de Tropen; 's-Gravenhage: NOVIB; Brussel NCOS, 1991.
2. Department of Economic and Social Development, Statistical Division. 1991 Demographic Yearbook. New York: United Nations, 1992.
3. World Bank. World Development Report 1993. Oxford: Oxford University Press, 1993.
4. Department of Economic and Social Information and Policy Analysis, Statistical Division. Statistical Yearbook 1990/91. Data vailable as of 1 September 1992. New York: United Nations, 1993.
5. UNICEF. The State of the World's Children. Oxford: Oxford University Press, 1993.
6. Mwaluko GMP, Kilama WL, Mandara MP, Murru M, MacPherson CNL. Health and Disease in Tanzania. London: Harper Collins Academic, 1991.
7. Klouda A. 'Prevention' is more costly than 'cure': health problems for Tanzania, 1971-81. In, Practicing health for all. Eds Morley D, Rohde J, Williams G. Oxford: Oxford University Press, 1983.
8. Bryant J. Health and the developing world. Ithaka: Cornell University Press, 1969.
9. Robinson D. Epidemiology and the community control of disease in warm climate countries. London: Churchill Livingstone, 1985.
10. Global Programme on AIDS. Global strategy for the prevention and control of AIDS: 1992 update. WHA45/29. Geneva: World Health Organization, 1992.
11. Van Roosmalen J. Maternal health care in the South Western highlands of Tanzania. Leiden: PhD thesis, 1988.
12. Van Roosmalen-Wiebenga MW. Nutrition rehabilitation in the South Western highlands of Tanzania. A two way learning process. Amsterdam: PhD thesis, 1988.
13. Barongo LR, Borgdorff MW, Mosha FF, et al. The prevalence of HIV infection, syphilis, and STD syndromes in Mwanza Region. Unpublished research report. Mwanza: National Institute for Medical Research, 1991.
14. National AIDS Control Programme. HIV/AIDS/STD surveillance. Report No 7. Dar es Salaam: Ministry of Health, 1992.
15. National AIDS Control Programme, Tanzania. Strategic plan for Medium Term Plan II for AIDS control 1992-1996. Dar es Salaam: Ministry of Health, 1992.
16. Dolmans WMV, Van Loon AM, Van den Akker R, et al. Prevalence of HIV-1 antibody among groups of patients and healthy subjects from a rural and urban population in the Mwanza Region, Tanzania. AIDS 1989;3:297-299.
17. Van den Akker R, Bouman-van Engelen CAA, De Jong JC, et al. Persistence of anti-p24 antibodies in African AIDS patients. AIDS 1988;2:62-63.
18. Dolmans WMV, Van den Akker R, Van Loon AM, et al. HIV-infectie en AIDS in de Mwanza Regio, Tanzania: een voorstudie. Ned Tijdschr Geneesk 1989;133:1811.
19. Velema JP, Van Asten HGAG, Klokke AH, et al. Vergelijking van de kwaliteit van snelle testen voor het bepalen van de HIV-status van bloeddonoren onder veldomstandigheden in Afrika. Tijdschrift voor Sociale Geneeskunde 4/92:38.
20. Dolmans WMV, Klokke AH, Van Asten HGAG, et al. Prevention of HIV transmission through blood transfusion in Tanzania. Trop Geogr Med 1992;44:285.
21. Barongo LR, Borgdorff MW, Mosha FF, et al. The epidemiology of HIV-1 infection in urban areas, roadside settlements and rural villages in Mwanza Region, Tanzania. AIDS 1992;6:1521-1528.
22. Mosha F, Nicoll A, Barongo L, et al. A population-based study of syphilis and sexually transmitted

disease syndromes in north-western Tanzania. 1. Prevalence and incidence. Genitourinary Medicine 1993;69:415-420.

23. Newell J, Senkoro K, Mosha F, et al. A population-based study of syphilis and sexually transmitted disease syndromes in north-western Tanzania. 2. Risk factors and health seeking behaviour. Genitourinary Medicine 1993;69:421-426.

24. Borgdorff M, Barongo L, Jaarsveld E van, et al. Sentinel surveillance for HIV-1 infection: How representative are blood donors; outpatients with fever, anaemia, or sexually transmitted diseases; and antenatal clinic attenders in Mwanza Region, Tanzania? AIDS 1993;7:567-572.

25. Kigadye RM, Klokke A, Nicoll A, et al. Sentinel surveillance for HIV-1 among pregnant women in a developing country: 3 years experience and comparison with a population survey. AIDS 1993;7:849-855.

26. Barongo LR, Borgdorff MW, Newell JN, et al. Intake of a cohort study of urban factory workers in northwest Tanzania: risk factors for HIV-1 infection. Trop Geograph Med 1994;46:157-162.

27. Borgdorff MW, Barongo LR, Newell JN, et al. Sexual partner change and condom use among urban factory workers in northwest Tanzania. Genitourin Med 1994 (in press).

28. Borgdorff MW, Barongo LR, Klokke AH, et al. HIV-1 incidence and HIV-1 associated mortality and morbidity in a cohort of urban factory workers in northwest Tanzania. (Submitted for publication).

29. Broek J van den, Borgdorff MW, Pakker NG, et al. HIV-1 infection as a risk factor for the development of tuberculosis disease: a population-based case-control study in Tanzania. Int J Epidemiol 1993;22:1159-1165.

30. Borgdorff MW, Broek J van den, Chum H, et al. HIV-1 infection as a risk factor for leprosy: a case-control study in Tanzania. Int J Leprosy 1993;61:556-562.

31. Nnko S, Mwanga J, Varkevisser C, et al. Risk perception and behavioural change in relation to AIDS. An exploratory study among factory workers in Mwanza town, Tanzania. In, Action research for the development of interventions to reduce HIV transmission in Mwanza Region, Tanzania. Amsterdam: KIT Press (in press).

32. Gumodoka B, Vos J, Kigadye FC, Van Asten H, Dolmans WMV, Borgdorff MW. Blood transfusion practices in Mwanza Region, Tanzania. AIDS 1993;7:387-392.

33. Vos J, Gumodoka B, Ng'weshemi JZL, Kigadye FC, Dolmans WMV, Borgdorff MW. Are some blood transfusion avoidable? A hospital record analysis in Mwanza Region, Tanzania. Tropical and Geographical Medicine 1993;45:301-303.

34. Vos J, Gumodoka B, van Asten HA, Berege ZA, Dolmans WM, Borgdorff MW. Changes in blood transfusion practices after the introduction of consensus guidelines in Mwanza Region, Tanzania. AIDS 1994; 8:1135-1140.

35. Gumodoka B, Vos J, Berege ZA, van Asten HA, Dolmans WM, Borgdorff MW. Injection practices increasing risk of HIV transmission in Mwanza Region, Tanzania: prescriptions, patient demand and sterility. (Submitted for publication)

36. Vos J, Gumodoka B, Van Asten HAGH, Berege ZA, Dolmans WMV, Borgdorff MW. Changes in injection practices after the introduction of treatment and sterility guidelines. (In preparation).

3

The epidemiology of HIV-1 infection in urban areas, roadside settlements and rural villages in Mwanza Region, Tanzania

Longin R. Barongo[1], Martien W. Borgdorff[1,2], Frank F. Mosha[1], Angus Nicoll[3,4], Heiner Grosskurth[3,4], Kesheni P. Senkoro[1], James N. Newell[1,3,4], John Changalucha[1], Arnoud H. Klokke[5], Japhet Z. Killewo[6], Johan P. Velema[7], Richard J. Hayes[4], David T. Dunn[4], Lex A.S. Muller[2], Joas B. Rugemalila[1]

AIDS 1992; 6:1521-1528

Summary

Objective: To determine the prevalence of HIV-1 infection and to identify the most important risk factors for infection.

Design: A cross-sectional population survey carried out in 1990 and 1991 in Mwanza Region, Tanzania.

Methods: Adults aged 15–54 years were selected from the region (population, 2 million) by stratified random cluster sampling: 2434 from 20 rural villages, 1157 from 20 roadside settlements and 1554 from 20 urban wards. Risk factor information was obtained from interviews. All sera were tested for HIV-1 antibodies using enzyme-linked immunosorbent assay (ELISA); sera non-negative on ELISA were also tested by Western blot.

Results: The response rate was 81%. HIV-1 infection was 1.5 times more common in women than in men; 2.5% of the adult population in rural villages, 7.3% in roadside settlements and 11.8% in town were infected. HIV-1 infection occurred mostly in women aged 15–34 years and men aged 25–44 years. It was associated with being separated or widowed, multiple sex partners, presence of syphillis antibodies, history of genital discharge or genital ulcer, travel to Mwanza town, and receiving injections during the previous 12 months, but not with male circumcision.

Conclusion: This study confirms that HIV-1 infection in this region in East Africa is more common in women than in men. The results are consistent with the spread of HIV-1 infection along the main roads. There is no evidence that lack of circumcision is a risk factor in this polulation.

[1] National Institute for Medical Research, Mwanza, Tanzania
[2] Royal Tropical Institute, Amsterdam, The Netherlands
[3] AMREF, Mwanza, Tanzania
[4] London School of Hygiene and Tropical Medicine, London, U.K.
[5] Bugando Medical Centre, Mwanza, Tanzania
[6] Muhimbili Medical Centre, Dept of Epidemiology, Dar es Salaam, Tanzania
[7] Institute for Health care in Developing Countries, Nijmegen, The Netherlands

Introduction

Approximately half of the reported AIDS cases in Africa originate from East Africa (Uganda, Kenya, Tanzania, Rwanda, and Burundi) [1]. There is a large variation in the prevalence of HIV-1 within East Africa, as shown by general population surveys [2-4] and tests on selected groups [5,6]. Seroprevalence is generally high in towns and lower in rural areas. Within Tanzania, some regions, such as Kagera and Dar es Salaam, are much more affected than others [7]. It has been suggested that HIV-1 infection could spread along the trade routes in East Africa [4,8]. Main roads connecting Kenya, Rwanda, Burundi, Kagera Region, and Dar es Salaam pass through Mwanza Region, which is on the shores of Lake Victoria in northwestern Tanzania and has a population of approximately 2 million.

This region-wide population survey was undertaken between August 1990 and February 1991 to determine the prevalence of HIV-1 infection and other sexually transmitted diseases (STD), and to identify important risk factors. The findings on other STD will be reported elsewhere. The survey was conducted in preparation for further longitudinal and intervention studies in this region.

Methods

Each household within Tanzania belongs to a 10-cell unit, a subdivision within the hierarchical political organization of the country. Ten-cell units are composed of approximately 10 households and aggregated to form villages (or wards within the Mwanza Municipality) these are aggregated to form districts. This organization provides a well-defined and convenient structure for use in cluster sampling.

For this study, Mwanza Region was divided into three strata: urban, roadside and rural. The urban stratum consisted of Mwanza Municipality, the roadside stratum of the small towns and villages through which the main roads to Kenya, Rwanda, Burundi, Kagera Region and Dar es Salaam pass, and the rural stratum of all other villages.

To obtain HIV-1 prevalence estimates of adequate precision, calculations indicated that sample sizes of at least 2000 from the rural stratum, and 1000 from each of the roadside and urban strata, would be required. This was achieved by randomly selecting 20 villages (or wards) from each stratum, with the probability of selection proportional to the size of the village (ward) population. The population data came from the 1978 census for the rural and roadside strata and from the 1988 census for the urban stratum; these provided the most recent data available at the time of the survey. Within selected villages and wards, 10-cell units were selected using simple random sampling from a listing of all 10-cell units, to give an average total of 100 eligible individuals, aged 15–54 years, in each rural site (usually from three to four 10-cell units), and 50 eligible individuals, aged 15–54 years in each roadside and urban site (usually from two 10-cell units). The aim was to survey all eligible individuals in the selected 10-cell units, a list of whom had been prepared by the chairman of the 10-cell unit before the survey. Because of variability in the size of 10-cell units, the final numbers selected for inclusion in the rural, roadside and urban strata were 2434, 1157, and 1554 respectively.

Local communities were approached through the regional authorities and through the government and party leaders in all six districts, and in the wards and villages selected. Informed (oral) consent was obtained. The community was told that the study was a survey of STD, including HIV-1 infection, and that those found to have treatable STD, such as syphilis or genital discharge would receive treatment. HIV-1 testing was anonymous, using code numbers in accordance with Tanzanian government guidelines on HIV-1 testing. Individuals wishing to know their HIV-1 test result were asked to give a separate, named, blood sample, and were referred for pre- and postresult counselling to the district health services.

Respondents were interviewed at a convenient central location in the village (ward) such as the party office, by a trained interviewer of the same sex, using a pre-coded questionnaire; each interview lasted approximately 20 minutes. Between 5–10 ml venous blood was taken, using a vacuum system, and the blood sample separated in the field. Those reporting the presence of a genital ulcer or discharge were examined clinically by a physician. The physicians' findings were not used to reclassify responses to the questionnaire.

Non-respondents were visited at home and encouraged to participate. Reasons for continued non-response, such as refusal or absence from home, were recorded. The final number of respondents in the rural, roadside and urban strata were 2024, 962 and 1187, with response rates of 83, 83 and 76%, respectively. Response rates were not associated with sex or age group.

Serum was tested for HIV-1 antibodies using the Vironostika enzyme-linked immuno-sorbent assay (ELISA; Organon, Boxtel, The Netherlands). All non-negative samples underwent confirmatory testing using Western blot (Organon; Epitope, Beaverton, Oregon, USA). Western blot was considered positive if at least two of the gp41, gp120, and gp160 bands were present [9]. Indeterminate blot results were classed as negative in the analysis. A Treponema pallidum haemagglutination test (TPHA; Fujirebio, Tokyo, Japan) was performed to diagnose syphilis infection, followed by a rapid plasma reagin (RPR) test (VD-25; Wellcome, Dartford, England, UK) on sera with a positive TPHA result. A positive TPHA with a positive RPR was interpreted as indicating active or recently treated syphilis infection, while a positive TPHA and negative RPR was interpreted as a cured syphilis infection [10].

For each of the three residential strata, and separately for men and women, weighted prevalences and confidence intervals (CI) were calculated for HIV-1 infection, for risk factors, and for HIV-1 infection within risk groups. Prevalences were corrected [11] to take account of the varying cluster sizes, although the effect of correction was small. Two estimates for odds ratios (OR) and their CI are presented: Mantel-Haenszel OR, adjusted for residential stratum, sex, and age; and OR obtained from logistic regression, adjusted for all significant factors. The effects of the cluster sampling scheme have been ignored in calculating the OR.

Figure I   HIV-I prevalence by age and residence in men and women

HIV prevalence males (%)

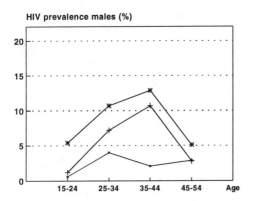

HIV prevalence females (%)

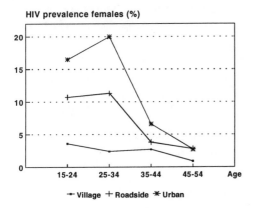

-*- Village -+- Roadside -*- Urban

Results

HIV-1 prevalence by age, sex, and residence
The prevalence of HIV-1 infection in rural villages, roadside settlements and urban wards was 2.5% (95% CI, 1.7-3.7), 7.3% (CI, 5.1-10.6), and 11.8% (CI, 9.5-14.7), respectively (Table 1). HIV-1 seroprevalence was higher in women than in men; the prevalence ratio was 1.2 in the rural, 1.6 in the roadside, and 1.7 in the urban stratum. Standardization by age group using the total study population as the standard population has little influence on these prevalence rates or on the female-to-male ratios. Women acquired HIV-1 infection at a younger age than men (Fig. 1); HIV-1 prevalence was highest in women aged 15–34 years and in men aged 25–44 years, with a peak of 20% in urban women aged 25–34 years.

Risk factors
Prevalences of HIV-1 infection by risk factor are presented in Table 2 for women, and in Table 3 for men. Adjusted OR for these associations are shown in Table 4.

Table 1. HIV-1 prevalence by age, sex and residence

Age (years)		No. (%)*		
		Village	Roadside	Urban
Men	15-24	2/ 314 (0.6)	2/ 134 (1.2)	12/ 222 (5.4)
	25-34	12/ 309 (4.0)	12/ 142 (7.2)	21/ 198 (10.7)
	35-44	4/ 191 (2.1)	8/ 84 (10.7)	15/ 116 (12.9)
	45-54	5/ 160 (2.9)	1/ 71 (2.8)	3/ 59 (5.1)
	Total	23/ 974 (2.4)	23/ 431 (5.4)	51/ 595 (8.7)
Women	15-24	14/ 397 (3.6)	18/ 183 (10.7)	38/ 245 (16.5)
	25-34	8/ 330 (2.4)	20/ 193 (11.3)	41/ 213 (20.0)
	35-44	5/ 210 (2.7)	3/ 83 (3.8)	8/ 86 (6.6)
	45-54	1/ 108 (0.9)	1/ 68 (2.8)	2/ 45 (2.7)
	Total	28/ 1045 (2.8)	42/ 527 (8.7)	89/ 589 (15.2)
Overall total		51/ 2019 (2.5)	65/ 958 (7.3)	140/ 1184 (11.8)
Female: male ratio		1.2	1.6	1.7
Design effects (rates of homogeneity)				
Men total		1.2 (0.004)	1.2 (0.010)	1.0 (0.001)
Women total		1.8 (0.016)	2.6 (0.063)	1.8 (0.028)
Overall total		2.0 (0.010)	2.9 (0.040)	2.0 (0.017)

* Percentages are weighted to take account of the cluster sampling scheme, so they are not identical to the unweighted percentages that can be calculated from this table.

In the rural and roadside strata, HIV-1 seroprevalence was higher in those who had travelled to Mwanza town in the previous 2 years. Prevalence was also higher in those who had moved to their present village or ward in that time, except in urban men. Travel outside the region was not a risk factor (data not shown).

After adjustment for age and residence, HIV-1 infection was not associated with educational level in either sex, or with occupation in men. Women who had an office job, or were employed in manual work or self-employed in business had a higher prevalence of HIV-1 infection than those who were farmers, housewives, or unemployed.

HIV-1 prevalence was higher in those who were separated, divorced or widowed than in those who were single or married, particularly in men. In women, this association disappeared on adjustment for reported number of partners, suggesting that the higher risk in separated, divorced or widowed women was attributable to a greater number of partners. There was a highly significant association between HIV-1 infection and reported number of sex partners in the previous 5 years in both sexes (test for trend adjusting for age, residence and other factors: $\chi^2=22.4$, p<0.001 for women; $\chi^2=5.8$, p=0.02 for men).

Table 2. Prevalence of HIV-1 infection by risk factor and residence in women

Risk factor	HIV prevalence (%)		
	Village	Roadside	Urban
Travel to Mwanza town in previous 2 years			
Yes	9/ 212 (4.5)	28/ 241 (12.8)	NA
No	17/ 817 (2.1)	14/ 286 (5.1)	NA
Moved in previous 2 years			
Yes	5/ 123 (4.9)	14/ 122 (13.1)	22/ 89 (25.0)
No	23/ 920 (2.5)	28/ 405 (7.5)	67/ 500 (13.3)
Education:			
≥4 years	18/ 433 (4.2)	33/ 315 (11.1)	61/ 407 (15.3)
<4 years	10/ 611 (1.8)	9/ 212(5:6)	28/ 180 (15.3)
Occupation			
Employed/ business	1/ 16 (6.1)	6/ 32 (23.4)	20/ 91 (20.7)
Farmer/ housewife	27/ 1008 (2.8)	36/ 488 (7.9)	65/ 472 (14.1)
Others	0/ 20 (0.0)	0/ 7 (0.0)	4/ 26 (13.7)
Marital status			
Separated/ widowed	6/ 152 (4.7)	11/ 118 (16.7)	22/ 86 (25.8)
Married	16/ 715 (2.2)	16/ 310 (4.9)	35/ 351 (13.3)
Single	4/ 166 (2.4)	10/ 97 (11.5)	17/ 116 (14.3)
Partners in previous 5 years (n)			
Two or more	7/ 183 (3.9)	15/ 147 (11.9)	45/ 169 (26.3)
One	20/ 703 (3.0)	27/ 348 (8.3)	35/ 351 (10.2)
None	1/ 122 (0.7)	0/ 32 (0.0)	9/ 69 (11.4)
Genital ulcer ever			
Yes	2/ 45 (2.7)	4/ 29 (17.9)	3/ 18 (20.5)
No	26/ 1000 (4.4)	38/ 498 (8.3)	86/ 583 (15.1)
Genital discharge ever			
Yes	5/ 82 (6.1)	0/ 30 (0.0)	10/ 28 (32.9)
No	23/ 963 (2.5)	42/ 497 (9.3)	79/ 561 (14.4)
Syphilis now			
Yes	4/ 81 (5.0)	7/ 67 (11.7)	15/ 68 (23.2)
No	23/ 963 (2.6)	35/ 460 (8.4)	74/ 520 (14.1)
Syphilis ever			
Yes	6/ 140 (4.4)	9/ 114 (9.6)	27/ 123 (21.4)
No	22/ 906 (2.5)	33/ 414 (8.6)	62/ 467 (13.6)
Injection(s) in previous 12 months			
One or more	17/ 595 (2.9)	32/ 300 (12.2)	62/ 361 (16.9)
None	11/ 448 (2.6)	10/ 227 (4.4)	27/ 228 (12.4)

Notes: Percentages are weighted to take account of the cluster sampling scheme. Explanation of categories: moved previous 2 years – from another village or ward; those with occupation 'other' were mainly school children; number of partners in previous 5 years – question was on 'number of formal and informal marriages in previous 5 years'; 'ever' included now for sexually transmitted disease syndromes. NA, not applicable.

Table 3.   Prevalence of HIV-1 infection by risk factor and residence in men

Risk factor	HIV prevalence (%)		
	Village	Roadside	Urban
Travel to Mwanza town in previous 2 years			
Yes	13/ 388 (3.3)	18/ 289 (6.1)	NA
No	9/ 571 (1.6)	5/ 142 (4.0)	NA
Moved in previous 2 years			
Yes	6/ 64 (9.4)	5/ 43 (10.4)	6/ 133 (4.2)
No	17/ 909 (1.8)	18/ 388 (4.9)	45/ 462 (9.8)
Education:			
≥4 years	15/ 682 (2.2)	22/ 326 (6.9)	44/ 523 (8.5)
<4 years	8/ 290 (2.6)	1/ 105 (0.9)	7/ 72 (9.6)
Occupation			
Employed/ business	2/ 77 (2.4)	8/ 102 (6.3)	31/ 340 (8.6)
Farmer	20/ 850 (2.3)	15/ 297 (5.6)	16/ 193 (9.1)
Other	1/ 45 (2.8)	0/ 31 (0.0)	4/ 62 (7.7)
Marital status			
Separated/ widowed	10/ 83 (11.5)	5/ 47 (9.7)	10/ 49 (20.4)
Married	9/ 621 (1.4)	15/ 258 (6.3)	30/ 309 (9.7)
Single	3/ 253 (1.2)	3/ 125 (1.8)	11/ 236 (4.8)
Partners in previous 5 years (n)			
Two or more	14/ 442 (3.2)	19/ 264 (6.8)	42/ 425 (9.9)
One	6/ 359 (1.5)	4/ 135 (3.9)	9/ 142 (6.9)
None	3/ 150 (2.0)	0/ 32 (0.0)	0/ 28 (0.0)
Genital ulcer ever			
Yes	4/ 142 (3.0)	5/ 66 (7.0)	15/ 97 (16.4)
No	19/ 830 (2.2)	18/ 365 (5.1)	36/ 498 (7.2)
Genital discharge ever			
Yes	10/ 268 (3.8)	13/ 130 (10.3)	32/ 185 (16.8)
No	13/ 706 (1.8)	10/ 301 (3.4)	19/ 410 (5.0)
Syphilis now			
Yes	1/ 67 (2.2)	7/ 48 (15.9)	8/ 55 (13.2)
No	22/ 905 (2.4)	16/ 383 (3.9)	43/ 539 (8.2)
Syphilis ever			
Yes	2/ 127 (1.6)	9/ 92 (10.8)	15/ 95 (13.9)
No	21/ 851 (2.4)	14/ 342 (3.8)	36/ 502 (7.6)
Circumcision			
Yes	4/ 159 (2.4)	6/ 132 (4.0)	32/351 (9.8)
No	19/ 813 (2.3)	17/ 299 (6.0)	19/ 244 (6.8)
Injection (s)in previous 12 months			
One or more	12/ 388 (3.1)	12/ 167 (6.7)	34/ 302 (11.0)
None	11/ 586 (1.8)	11/ 264 (4.5)	17/ 293 (6.2)

Percentages are weighted to take account of the cluster sampling scheme. Explanation of categories: moved previous 2 years – from another village or ward; those with occupation 'other' were mainly school children; number of partners in previous 5 years – question was on 'number of formal and informal marriages in previous 5 years'; 'ever' included now for sexually transmitted disease syndromes. NA, not applicable.

Table 4. Odds ratios (OR) of risk factors for HIV-1 infection in men and women (1) adjusted for age and residence stratum, and (2) adjusted for factors of interest using logistic regression

Risk factor	OR adjusted for age and residence (95%CI)		OR adjusted for factors of interest* using logistic regression	
	Women	Men	Women	Men
Travel to Mwanza town in previous 2 years	2.1 (1.2-3.6)	1.7 (0.8-3.5)	1.7 (1.0-2.9)	1.3 (0.7-2.6)
Moved in previous 2 years	1.8 (1.2-2.7)	1.1 (0.6-2.0)	1.4 (0.9-2.1)	1.0 (0.5-1.8)
≥4 years education	1.1 (0.8-1.7)	1.2 (0.7-2.3)	1.2 (0.8-1.9)	1.1 (0.6-2.0)
OccupationE				
Employed/business	2.0 (1.2-3.4)	1.1 (0.6-1.8)	1.5 (0.9-2.6)	0.9 (0.6-1.6)
Other (non-farming)	0.7 (0.2-2.2)	1.2 (0.4-3.7)	0.8 (0.3-2.6)	1.3 (0.5-3.6)
Marital status				
Separated/widowed	2.1 (1.0-4.5)	5.9 (2.9-12.1)	1.6 (0.9-3.0)	3.4 (1.6-7.6)
Married	1.0 (0.6-1.7)	1.7 (0.9-3.1)	0.6 (0.3-1.1)	1.0 (0.5-2.1)
Partners in previous 5 years (n)				
Two or more	3.7 (1.6-8.9)	1.6 (0.4-7.1)	3.6 (1.6-8.2)	2.3 (0.5-10.4
One	1.7 (0.8-3.8)	0.9 (0.2-5.3)	2.0 (0.9-4.6)	1.4 (0.3-6.6)
Genital ulcer ever	1.6 (0.7-3.5)	1.6 (0.9-2.7)	1.1 (0.5-2.5)	1.1 (0.7-1.9)
Genital discharge ever	2.0 (1.1-3.7)	2.7 (1.8-4.3)	1.7 (0.9-2.5)	2.2 (1.4-3.5)
Syphilis now	1.7 (1.0-2.7)	1.9 (1.0-3.5)	1.2 (0.6-2.5)	1.3 (0.6-3.2)
Syphilis ever	1.7 (1.1-2.5)	1.8 (1.0-2.9)	1.5 (1.0-2.3)	1.5 (0.9-2.4)
Circumcision	NA	0.9 (0.6-1.5)	NA	0.8 (0.5-1.3)
One or more injections in previous 12 months	1.5 (1.1-2.2)	1.9 (1.2-2.9)	1.5 (1.0-2.2)	1.7 (1.1-2.7)

* Factors adjusted for in logistic regression: age group, residence stratum, travel to Mwanza town, marital status, number of partners, genital discharge ever, syphilis ever, injection in previous 12 months. The baseline OR of 1 is given to those without the risk factor under consideration. CI, confidence interval; NA, not applicable.

HIV-1 prevalence was higher in those reporting that they had ever had a genital discharge or ulcer, in both sexes. The association with history of genital ulcer disappeared on adjustment for number of partners, while the association with history of discharge was weakened but still significant in men. In rural villages, roadside settlements and urban areas, a positive TPHA was found in 13.3, 22.0, and 18.1% of the adult population, respectively; untreated or recently treated syphilis was found in 7.4, 12.6 and 10.4%, respectively. HIV-1 infection was associated with serological evidence of past or present syphilis in both sexes (Table 4). This association remained significant on adjustment for number of partners in women.

There was no evidence of any association between HIV-1 infection and male circumcision, before or after adjustment for other risk factors. HIV-1 infection was more common among those who had received one or more injections from medical staff in the previous 12 months, particularly in men.

The role of some potential risk factors could not be assessed. Contraceptives, including condoms, were used by so few people (condoms, 2.5%; herbs, 2.1%; others, 2.5%) that it was not possible to determine their association with HIV-1 infection in this survey. Injections by practitioners without medical training were reported too infrequently (by fewer than 5% of respondents) for statistical analysis, although it appears likely that these were under-reported. Since very few people reported receiving blood transfusions (2.1%), their association with HIV-1 infection in this population remains unclear.

Discussion

The prevalence rate of HIV-1 infection was high in town (11.8%), much lower in rural villages (2.5%), and intermediate in roadside settlements (7.3%). This is consistent with the suggested spread of the infection along African main roads [4,8].
Since the estimated 1990 population (aged 15-54 years) of Mwanza Region in rural villages, roadside settlements, and urban areas was 637,000, 139,000, and 132,000, respectively, the total number of HIV-1 infected adults in the Region can be estimated to be approximately 42,000, indicating an overall adult prevalence of 4.6%. Of all adults with HIV-1 infection, approximately 40% live in Mwanza Municipality, 20% in roadside settlements, and another 40% in rural areas. HIV-1 infection is often regarded as primarily a problem of urban populations [12]. While prevalence rates are certainly higher in urban areas, in Mwanza Region (as in many African countries) the majority of people live in rural areas, so there are as many people with HIV-1 infection in rural villages as in Mwanza Municipality. Although AIDS control efforts in towns may be more cost-effective, rural areas should not be neglected.

Selection of the villages was based on 1978 census data, since data from the 1988 census were available only for Mwanza Municipality. Although demographic changes are likely to be largest between strata (people moving from rural to urban areas), there will also have been some migration within each stratum. Thus, faster growing villages and roadside settlements are likely to have been under-reported in this survey, which may have led to a slight underestimation of HIV-1 prevalence.

Although we consider a coverage of 76–83% in the three strata to be a reasonable accomplishment, we expect that HIV-1 prevalence in non-attenders was somewhat higher than in attenders, because people who travel frequently are likely to be at increased risk of HIV-1 infection and were more likely to be absent at the time of the survey. Therefore, it seems reasonable to expect that incomplete coverage caused an underestimation of HIV-1 prevalence. We expect this bias to be small because response rates were not associated with sex or age group.

It is unclear whether seroprevalence is higher in towns because HIV-1 infection was introduced earlier, or because risk behaviour is different. The former is very likely to be the case, but the latter may also play a role. Social control is stronger in villages, and it appears likely that this reduces the risk of HIV-1 infection. This is reflected in a number of risk factors. For example, in rural villages a smaller proportion of people reported more than one sex partner in the previous 5 years than in roadside settlements or in town. Similarly, fewer people had an untreated or recently treated syphilis infection in the rural villages.

The importance of mobility is shown in the rural and roadside strata by the increased HIV-1 prevalence in those who had travelled to town or moved to their present village during the previous 2 years. Travel outside the region was not associated with increased risk, possibly because HIV-1 infection is less common in some areas than others in Mwanza Region.

Approximately half of notified AIDS cases in Tanzania and Uganda, are women [7,13]. In our study HIV-1 prevalence in women was 1.2–1.7 times greater than in men, depending on the residential stratum: the sex difference was clearest in towns. Similar results have been reported from Kagera Region [3], Rwanda [2] and Uganda [4,14]. The observed difference may be partly artefactual because of sampling bias. Mobile men, who are at high risk, are more likely not to be included in this type of survey. However, if sampling bias were the only explanation for the observed sex difference, HIV-1 prevalence in absentees would have to be very much higher in men than in women. Therefore, a real difference appears likely, and this may be due to a greater efficiency of HIV-1 transmission from men to women than from women to men. This would be consistent with the results of some studies on spouses of HIV-1 infected individuals [15,16].

The age distribution of HIV-1 infected men and women is as expected from the age distribution of notified AIDS cases [7,13]. In general, HIV-1 infection is most prevalent among women aged 15-34 and men aged 25–44 years. The high prevalence in women in this age group is of particular concern, because of the possibility of transmission of the virus to offspring during pregnancy.

The high prevalence of HIV-1 in separated, divorced, and widowed individuals has also been found in studies in Zaire and The Gambia [17,18]. Possible explanations are an increased likelihood of separation among people with multiple partners, and an increased likelihood of having multiple partners among people who are separated. The question asked in our study about the number of partners in the previous 5 years had limited validity. It was worded vaguely to avoid embarrassment ('How many *formal* and *informal* marriages did you have in the previous 5 years'), and is likely to have been interpreted differently by each respondent and interviewer. Despite these problems, HIV-1 prevalence was clearly associated with reported number of partners in both sexes. However, for an accurate description of the epidemiology of STD, including HIV-1 infection, more detailed information on the number and type of partners is clearly needed. It is unlikely that this information can be obtained reliably from a survey of this type, because of problems of definition, embarrassment and recall.

We were unable to find any evidence of an association between the absence of circumcision in men and HIV-1 infection, although a moderate protective effect cannot be excluded (adjusted OR, 0.8; 95% CI, 0.5-1.3). Given a true association, misclassification would disguise the effect; however, subsequent work at an urban STD clinic in the Region showed that men invariably reported their circumcision status correctly. Although an association has been suggested by studies on STD clinic attenders in Nairobi [19,20] and by reviews of data on the prevalence of HIV-1 infection and of circumcision in various countries and regions [21,22], this has not been confirmed by others [23]. Since circumcision is associated with factors such as lifestyle and religion, the association reported by others, or the lack of association found in this study, may be due to confounding. In our study, for example, circumcision was more common in town (61%) than in roadside settlements (29%) or rural villages (17%). It is not practiced widely in rural areas and is not a traditional custom. Those who are circumcised are therefore more likely to be urban, mobile, and 'modern' (i.e., not strongly tied to traditional customs). Any protective effect of circumcision may not be obvious because it occurs within a group that is at increased risk of HIV-1 infection. On the other hand, the association shown in STD clinic attenders [19,20] may similarly be due to confounding. In the two reviews referred to above [21,22], populations rather than indivisuals were compared, and confounding could not be controlled for at all. A longitudinal study that we have started in the same region may provide more conclusive evidence, both on the possible protective role offered by circumcision, and on various sexual behaviour patterns as risk factors for HIV-1 infection.

The comparatively weak association found between HIV-1 and syphilis serology may result from many people acquiring syphilis at a time when the risk of HIV-1 infection was still very low. Measurement inaccuracies in reported STD syndromes are likely to be large: there was only a limited association between reported STD syndromes and findings on clinical examination. This was particularly the case for women. Despite these measurement problems, an association between HIV-1 infection and a history of genital discharge was observed, even after allowing for number of sex partners. Intervention studies are needed to establish that this association is causal [24]; one such has just started in Mwanza Region.

The higher prevalence of HIV-1 in those reporting one or more injections in the previous 12 months is in accordance with the findings of others [8,25,26]. The association between HIV-1 infection and receiving injections may be confounded by treatment for those STD that were not reported in the interviews. If the association is real, it has two probable explanations. First, HIV-1 infected people are more likely to require medical treatment, including injections. Secondly, some transmission of HIV-1 may have occurred via unsterilized needles or syringes.

A number of conclusions may be drawn for preventive interventions. Target groups should include adolescents, particularly women. Priority intervention areas are towns and roadside settlements, although villages should not be neglected. Condom use needs to be promoted more strongly and strategies aiming at the reduction of partner-change need to be developed urgently. As a follow-up to this study, a programme for the control of STD is being introduced in the region, as are measures to reduce the number of unnecessary injections and to improve sterilization practices.

Acknowledgements

We thank the Principal Secretary, Ministry of Health, and the Director-General of the National Institute for Medical Research, Dar es Salaam, Tanzania, for permission to carry out and publish the results of this study. Support of regional, district, ward, and village government and party officials is gratefully acknowledged. We are particularly grateful for the support and hospitality of the people included in the survey. We thank Prof. R.A. Coutinho for critically reviewing the manuscript.

Sponsorship: Financed by Netherlands Minister for Development Cooperation, (Dept DST/SO) and EC AIDS Task Force. Salary support from Wellcome Trust (A.N.) and Overseas Development Administratiion (A.N. and H.G.).

References

1. World Health Organization: Acquired immune deficiency syndrome - Data as at 31 January 1991. Wkly Epidemiol Rec 1991, 66:25-26.
2. Rwandan HIV Seroprevalence Study Group: Nationwide community-based serological survey of HIV-1 and other human retrovirus infections in a Central African country. Lancet 1989, i:941-943.
3. Killewo J, Nyamuryekunge K, Sandström a, et al: Prevalence of HIV-1 infection in the Kagera region of Tanzania: a population-based study. AIDS 1990, 4:1081-1085.
4. Wawer MJ, Serwadda D, Musgrave SD, Konde-Lulu JK, Musagara M, Sewankambo NK: Dynamics of spread of HIV-1 infection in a rural district of Uganda. BMJ 1991, 303:1303-1306.
5. Mhalu F, Bredberg-Radén U, Mbena E, et al: Prevalence of HIV infection in healthy subjects and groups of patients in Tanzania. AIDS 1987, 1:217-221.
6. Dolmans WMV, Van Loon AM, Van den Akker R, et al: Prevalence of HIV-1 antibody among groups of patients and healthy subjects from a rural and urban population in the Mwanza region, Tanzania. AIDS 1989, 3:297-299.
7. Ministry of Health. National AIDS Control Programme: AIDS Surveillance. Report No. 4. Dar es Salaam: Epidemiology Unit NACP, 1991.
8. Carswell JW, Lloyd G, Howells J: Prevalence of HIV-1 in East African lorry drivers. AIDS 1989, 3:759-761.
9. World Health Organization: Acquired immune deficiency syndrome (AIDS) - proposed WHO criteria for interpreting results from Western blot assays for HIV-1, HIV-2, and HTLV-I/HTLV-II. Wkly Epidemiol Rec 1990, 65:281-283.

10. Adler MW: ABC of sexually transmitted diseases. London: British Medical Association, 1984.

11. Bennett S, Woods AJ, Liyanage WM, Smith DL: A simplified general method for cluster sample surveys of health in developing countries. World Health Statistics Quarterly 1991, 44:98-105.

12. Piot P, Plummer FA, Mhalu FS, Lamboray JL, Chin J, Mann JM: AIDS: an international perspective. Science 1988, 239:573-579.

13. Berkley S, Okware S, Naamara W: Surveillance for AIDS in Uganda. AIDS 1989, 3:79-85.

14. Berkley S, Naamara W, Okware S, et al: AIDS and HIV infection in Uganda - are more women infected than men? AIDS 1990, 4:1237-1242.

15. Laga M, Taelman H, Van der Stuyft P, Bonneux L, Vercauteren G, Piot P: Advanced immunodeficiency as a risk factor for heterosexual transmission of HIV. AIDS 1989, 3:361-366.

16. Johnson AM, Petherick A, Davidson SJ, et al: Transmission of HIV to heterosexual partners of infected men and women. AIDS 1989, 3:367-372.

17. Ryder RW, Ndilu M, Hassig SE, et al: Heterosexual transmission of HIV-1 among employees and their spouses at two large businesses in Zaire. AIDS 1990, 4:725-732.

18. Wilkins A, Hayes R, Alonso P, et al: Risk factors for HIV-2 infection in The Gambia. AIDS 1991, 5:1127-1132.

19. Cameron DW, Simonsen JN, D'Costa LJ, et al: Female-to-male transmission of human immunodeficiency virus type 1: risk factors for seroconversion in men. Lancet 1989, ii:403-407.

20. Simonsen JN, Cameron DW, Gakinya MN, et al: Human immunodeficiency virus infection among men with sexually transmitted diseases - experience from a center in Africa. New Engl J Med 1988, 319:274-278.

21. Bongaarts J, Reining P, Way P, Conant F: The relationship between male circumcision and HIV infection in African populations. AIDS 1989, 3:373-377.

22. Moses S, Bradley JE, Nagelkerke NJD, Ronald AR, Ndinya-Achola JD, Plummer FA: Geographical patterns of male circumcision practices in Africa: association with HIV seroprevalence. Int J Epidemiol 1990, 19:693-697.

23. Van de Perre P, Carael M, Nzaramba D, Zissis G, Kayihigi J, Butzler JP: Risk factors for HIV seropositivity in selected urban-based Rwandese adults. AIDS 1987, 1:207-211.

24. Mertens te, Hayes RJ, Smith PG: Epidemiological methods to study the interaction between HIV infection and other sexually transmitted diseases. AIDS 1990, 4:57-65.

25. Mann JM, Francis H, Davachi F, et al: Risk factors for human inmmunodeficiency virus seropositivity among children 1-24 months old in Kinshasa, Zaire. Lancet 1986, ii:654-657.

26. Mann JM, Francis H, Davachi F, et al: Human inmmunodeficiency virus seroprevalence in pediatric patients 2 to 14 years of age at Mama Yemo Hospital, Kinshasa, Zaire. Pediatrics 1986, 78:673-676.

4

Sentinel surveillance for HIV-1 infection: how representative are blood donors, outpatients with fever, anaemia, or sexually transmitted diseases, and antenatal clinic attenders in Mwanza Region, Tanzania?

Martien Borgdorff [1,5], *Longin Barongo* [1], *Ellen van Jaarsveld* [6], *Arnoud Klokke* [2], *Kesheni Senkoro* [1], *James Newell* [1,3,7], *Angus Nicoll* [3,7], *Frank Mosha* [1], *Heiner Grosskurth* [3,7], *Ronald Swai* [4], *Henri van Asten* [4], *Johan Velema* [6], *Richard Hayes* [7], *Lex Muller* [8] *and Joas Rugemalila* [1]

AIDS 1993; 7: 567-572

Summary

Objective: To assess the validity of extrapolation from sentinel data by comparing the HIV-1 prevalence of various sentinel groups with that of the general population in Mwanza Region, Tanzania.

Methods: In a population survey, 4161 individuals were selected in a stratified random cluster sample. Sentinel groups (all in the age group 15–54 years) included blood donors (n=1090); patients examined at district hospitals for the presence of malaria parasites (n=1488), anaemia (n=1339), or syphilis (n=33); and antenatal clinic attenders (n=1193). The HIV-1 serostatus of individuals selected from the population survey was tested using enzyme-linked immunosorbent assay (ELISA) and Western blot; 51% of the blood donors were tested using HIVCHEK, and all others using ELISA. HIV-1 prevalence was standardized for age, sex, and urban/non-urban location.

Results: HIV-1 prevalence (standardized by age, sex, and residence) in Mwanza Region was 4.0% (3.0% in non-urban areas and 11.3% in town). The standardized HIV-1 prevalences in the sentinel groups were: blood donors, 4.5%; patients with fever, 11.6%; patients with anaemia, 8.9%; urban sexually transmitted disease patients, 27.1%; urban antenatal clinic attenders, 11.8%. The crude prevalence in blood donors was 6.0%.

Conclusion: Blood donors who are related to blood recipients appear to be a representative sentinel group in this region, provided that data are standardized for age, sex, and urban/non-urban location. Patients with fever and antenatal clinic attenders may reflect trends, but data

1 National Institute for Medical Research, Mwanza, Tanzania
2 Bugando Medical Centre, Mwanza, Tanzania
3 AMREF, Mwanza, Tanzania
4 Ministry of Health, National AIDS Control Programme, Dar es Salaam, Tanzania
5 Royal Tropical Institute, Amsterdam, The Netherlands
6 Nijmegen Institute of International Health, Nijmegen, The Netherlands
7 London School of Hygiene and Tropical Medicine, London, UK
8 University of Amsterdam, The Netherlands

from patients with fever markedly overestimate, and data from antenatal clinic attenders under-estimate, population HIV-1 prevalence. Because self-selection of blood donors may become more pronounced, this comparison should be repeated later or elsewhere, should the opportunity arise.

Introduction

Current information on the prevalence of HIV-1 infection and its trend over time is important for planning AIDS control programmes. Although repeated population surveys could be used to provide this information, their cost is prohibitive in most countries. The World Health Organization has therefore recommended alternative sources of information, which are often referred to as sentinel systems [1]. Sentinel surveillance selects specific sites and population groups, and routinely tests a pre-determined number of individuals either continuously or at regular intervals. The main objectives of sentinel serosurveillance are to monitor trends and to provide a basis for evaluating preventive strategies [2,3]. A major limitation is that the representativeness of the groups tested is usually unknown: how comparable is the prevalence in sentinel groups with that of the general population or specific subgroups within that population? More importantly, how well do sentinel groups reflect trends in prevalence in the general population?

Mwanza Region is on the shores of Lake Victoria, northwest Tanzania, and has a population of approximately 2 million. Two sentinel groups have been used here since 1989: blood donors in all hospitals of the region, and antenatal clinic attenders in Mwanza Municipality. This study considered an additional group: outpatients from all six district hospitals who had given blood samples, usually for detection of malaria parasites or Haemoglobin (Hb) determination. A population survey to determine the prevalence of HIV-1 infection was performed in Mwanza Region between August 1990 and February 1991. This provided us with the opportunity to assess the current representativeness of the various groups used for sentinel surveillance.

Methods

Blood donors
Data on the prevalence of HIV-1 infection among blood donors have been collected since 1989 by the National AIDS Control Programme (NACP). A form containing infor-mation on age, sex, relationship of the donor to the recipient, HIV-1 test result, type of test used and name of hospital is completed for each blood donor; forms are sent from each hospital in the region to the Regional Medical Office every month, and from there to the NACP. To ensure confidentiality, there is no identifying information on the form. Computer entry is performed at the NACP. Blood donors are usually related to trans-fusion recipients, although some hospitals also use other donors, such as schoolchildren.

For January and February 1991, data were available on 1090 blood donors in the age group 15-54 years. Forty-nine per cent were tested using enzyme-immunosorbent assay

(ELISA) [Vironostika anti human T-cell lymphotropic virus (HTLV)-III; Organon Teknika, Boxtel, The Netherlands] and 51% with HIVChek (Dupont, Geneva, Switzerland).

To evaluate data entry errors, 244 (22%) of the original records were obtained from the Regional Medical Office, re-entered and a verification program run. Two errors (one in age; one in sex) were discovered and five HIV-1 results were missing and entered as negative.

Outpatients at district hospitals

Between October 1990 and March 1991 capillary blood samples were collected (on filter paper) from the first 800 outpatients in each of the district hospitals who had given blood samples for determining malaria parasitaemia, Hb determination, or, in Mwanza Municipality, syphilis serology at a clinic for sexually transmitted diseases (STD), which is part of the district hospital. The following data were recorded: hospital name, age and sex of the patient, and reason for taking blood. Patient names were not recorded. Code numbers were assigned to link the data recorded and the blood sample. Of the 4692 filter papers distributed, 4605 were returned with the accompanying forms to the referral hospital (Bugando Medical Centre), where they were tested as described elsewhere [4].

The analysis of dried blood samples collected on filter paper for HIV-1 antibodies has a high sensitivity and specificity [5,6]. It has been used extensively for HIV-1 sero-surveillance of newborns [7-10]. As a preliminary test for this study, capillary blood samples were collected on filter paper from 50 patients with a positive result and 50 with a negative result on HIV-1 ELISA analysis of venous blood. Immediate testing showed complete concordance. The filter papers were kept at room temperature for 4 months, after which the one sample with a previous indeterminate HIV-1 result tested negative. The other samples still showed complete concordance.

The following were excluded from the analysis: 981 individuals aged below 15 or over 54 years; 135 individuals of unknown age; 699 samples where the blood spots were too small to punch a fully soaked disk of 5 mm diameter; and 51 individuals with other variables missing (sex or reason for giving blood). The results are presented separately for patients with malaria slide, Hb determination, or syphilis serology: the 125 patients with both a malaria slide and Hb determination were included in both groups.

Antenatal clinic attenders

All pregnant women attending a central antenatal clinic in Mwanza Municipality for the first time during their pregnancy are routinely tested for anaemia and syphilis serology. The first 300 serum samples of each 3-month period are tested for HIV-1 antibodies using ELISA (Vironostika anti HTLV-III; Organon Teknika) after removing all identifying information, except age and parity. We have analysed data for 1193 women attending in the last half of 1990 and the first half of 1991.

Population survey

A full description of the survey, which took place between August 1990 and February 1991, is given elsewhere [11]. Mwanza Region was divided into three strata: urban, roadside and rural. The urban stratum comprised Mwanza Municipality, the roadside stratum the small towns and villages along the main roads, and the rural stratum all other villages. Twenty clusters were randomly selected from each of the urban, roadside and rural strata, giving a total of 1184, 958 and 2019 study participants aged between 15 and 54 years, respectively.

The age and sex of respondents and information on risk factors was recorded. Serum was tested for HIV-1 antibodies using ELISA (Vironostika anti HTLV-III; Organon Teknika). All non-negative samples were tested using Western blot (Organon Epitope, Beaverton, Oregon, USA).

Data analysis

HIV-1 prevalence by age group in the general population and sentinel groups was compared. Because residence was not recorded for sentinel groups, the health facility site was used to label sentinel groups as urban or non-urban. The overall comparisons between sentinel and survey data were performed after calculating standardized prevalence rates (using the 1978 census population as the standard) because the population survey data showed that HIV-1 infection was strongly associated with age, sex, and location. Standardized prevalence ratios were calculated as the ratio of the standardized prevalence rates in the sentinel group (P_s) and the general population (P_g). The standard error (s.e.) of this ratio (P_s/P_g) was calculated from:

$$\text{s.e. } (\log(P_s/P_g) = [\text{var}(P_s)/P_s2 + \text{var }(P_g)/P_g2]^{0.5}$$

and:

$$\text{var }(P_s) \Sigma \text{ w}_j2 \text{ d}_j \text{ (n}_j - \text{d}_j)/\text{n}_j3$$

where for each age/sex/residence stratum j, w_j is the proportion of the standard population in that stratum, n_j the number of people in the sentinel group, and d_j the number of HIV-infected people. var(P_g) is calculated in a similar manner. These formulae are derived from [12] with appropriate modifications to binomial variances.

Results

Table 1 shows the HIV-1 prevalence in the general population (as determined by the population survey) and in the sentinel groups. HIV-1 prevalences in the urban, roadside and rural strata were 11.8, 7.3 and 2.5%, respectively. HIV-1 infection was more common in women (affecting mainly those aged 15–34 years) than in men (affecting mainly those aged 25–44 years).

The crude HIV-1 prevalence in blood donors was 6% (65 out of 1090). The standardized HIV-1 prevalence (4.5%) was similar to that in the general population, in both the urban and non-urban areas (Table 2). HIV-1 prevalence by age group in blood donors was also similar to that in the general population (Fig. 1). In non-urban areas HIV-1 prevalence in men was higher ($P<0.05$), and that in women lower ($P>0.05$), than that in the general population. Blood donors were predominantly male. Thirty-two per cent (351 out of 1090) of blood donors were urban, while only 12% (79 963 out of 662 124) of the general population were urban. All blood donors were related to blood recipients.

Table 1. HIV-1 prevalence by age and sex in the general population and in five sentinel groups, Mwanza, Tanzania

Age group (years)		No. HIV+/total (%)			
		Urban		Non–urban	
		Male	Female	Male	Female
Population survey*	15–24	12/ 222 (5)	38/ 245 (17)	4/ 448 (1)	32/ 580 (5)
	25–34	21/ 198 (11)	41/ 213 (20)	24/ 351 (5)	28/ 523 (4)
	35–44	15/ 116 (13)	8/ 86 (7)	12/ 275 (3)	8/ 293 (3)
	45–54	3/ 59 (5)	2/ 45 (3)	6/ 231 (3)	2/ 176 (1)
	Total	51/ 595 (9)	89/ 589 (15)	46/ 1405 (3)	70/ 1572 (4)
Blood donors	15–24	8/ 103 (8)	3/ 8 (38)	5/ 163 (3)	1/ 76 (2)
	25–34	13/ 143 (9)	0/ 9 (0)	15/ 246 (6)	5/ 76 (7)
	35–44	7/ 68 (10)	0/ 2 (0)	5/ 108 (5)	0/ 20 (0)
	45–54	1/ 18 (6)	0/ 0 (–)	2/ 48 (4)	0/ 2 (0)
	Total	29/ 332 (9)	3/ 19 (16)	27/ 565 (5)	6/ 174 (3)
Outpatients with fever	15–24	9/ 100 (9)	24/ 126 (19)	10/ 131 (8)	25/ 296 (8)
	25–34	24/ 102 (24)	27/ 98 (28)	21/ 116 (18)	28/ 212 (13)
	35–44	8/ 40 (20)	7/ 35 (20)	10/ 66 (15)	7/ 83 (8)
	45–54	0/ 15 (0)	0/ 8 (0)	2/ 31 (6)	2/ 29 (7)
	Total	41/ 257 (16)	58/ 267 (22)	43/ 344 (13)	62/ 620 (10)
Outpatients with anaemia	15–24	0/ 3 (0)	1/ 13 (8)	4/ 66 (6)	52/ 636 (8)
	25–34	1/ 6 (17)	9/ 19 (47)	1/ 35 (3)	34/ 403 (8)
	35–44	0/ 0 (–)	1/ 4 (25)	7/ 23 (30)	3/ 96 (3)
	45–54	0/ 2 (0)	0/ 3 (0)	0/ 10 (0)	2/ 20 (10)
	Total	1/ 11 (9)	11/ 39 (28)	12/ 134 (9)	91/ 1155 (8)
STD clinic attenders	15–24	1/ 6 (17)	4/ 10 (40)	–	–
	25–34	4/ 9 (44)	2/ 4 (50)	–	–
	35–44	0/ 3 (0)	0/ 1 (0)	–	–
	45–54	0/ 0 (–)	0/ 0 (–)	–	–
	Total	5/ 18 (28)	6/ 15 (40)	–	–
Antenatal clinic attenders	15–24	–	64/ 648 (10)	–	–
	25–34	–	61/ 460 (13)	–	–
	35–44	–	13/ 85 (15)**	–	–
	45–54	–	– – **	–	–
	Total	–	138/ 1193 (12)	–	–

* Percentages for the population survey have been weighted to take account of the cluster sampling scheme. HIV–1 prevalence in non–urban areas was calculated as: (0.15 x roadside prevalence)+ (0.85 x rural prevalence). Fifteen per cent of the non–urban population lived in roadside settlements and 85% in rural villages.
** The age group recorded was >35 years. We have assumed that these participants were aged 35–44 years.

Figure 1. HIV-1 prevalence by sex, location, and age group in the general population, blood donors, patients at district hospitals with fever or anaemia, and urban antenatal clinic attenders. Table 1 shows the data supporting this figure. Sentinel groups of less than 100 people and subgroups of less than 10 people have been omitted

Urban males

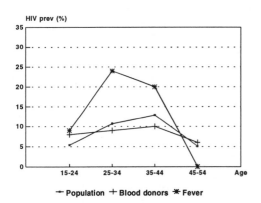

— Population + Blood donors ✳ Fever

Non-urban males

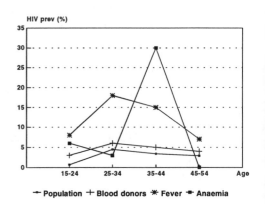

— Population + Blood donors ✳ Fever ✦ Anaemia

Urban females

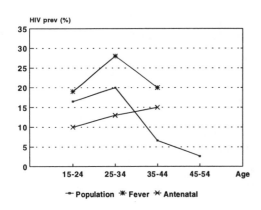

— Population ✳ Fever ✶ Antenatal

Non-urban females

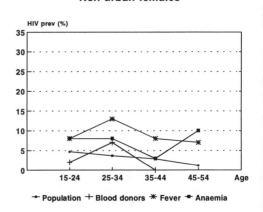

— Population + Blood donors ✳ Fever ✦ Anaemia

The crude HIV-1 prevalence in outpatients with fever who gave blood for a malaria slide 14% (204 out of 1488). The standardized HIV-1 prevalence in this group was markedly higher than in the general population, particularly in the non-urban area (Table 2). HIV-1 prevalence by age was consistently higher in this group than in the general population (Fig. 1). Thirty-five per cent (524 out of 1488) of outpatients with fever giving blood for a malaria slide were urban, compared with only 12% of the general population.

Table 2. HIV-1 prevalence in sentinel groups in urban and non–urban areas compared to HIV-1 prevalence in the general population, Mwanza, Tanzania

	HIV–1 prevalence(%)		Standardized prevalence ratio (95% CI)**
	Crude	Adjusted for age and sex*	
Population survey			
Urban	11.8	11.3	1
Non–urban	3.2	3.0	1
Total	–	4.0	1
Blood donors			
Urban	9.1	12.6	1.12 (0.62–2.02)
Non–urban	4.5	3.4	1.11 (0.72–1.70)
Total	6.0	4.5	1.11 (0.79–1.58)
Outpatients			
Fever			
Urban	18.9	17.4	1.54 (1.21–1.96)
Non–urban	10.9	10.8	3.54 (2.68–4.66)
Total	13.7	11.6	2.86 (2.31–3.55)
Anaemia			
Urban	24.0	12.6	1.12 (0.59–2.10)
Non–urban	8.0	8.4	2.74 (1.91–3.94)
Total	8.6	8.9	2.20 (162–2.98)
Syphilis			
Urban	33.3	27.1	2.40 (1.46–3.94)
Antenatal clinic			
Urban	11.6	11.8	0.75 (0.58–0.98)

* Prevalences are also adjusted for urban/ non–urban differences for all totals and for age only for antenatal clinic attenders.

** The prevalence ratio is calculated as the standardized HIV-1 prevalence in the group indicated divided by the standardized HIV-1 prevalence from the population survey. In antenatal clinic attenders this ratio was calculated by dividing by the standardized HIV-1 prevalence in urban women aged 15–44 years (15.7%). CI, confidence interval.

The crude HIV-1 prevalence in outpatients examined for the presence of anaemia was 9% (115 out of 1339). Again, the standardized HIV-1 prevalence in this group was markedly higher than in the general population, particularly in the non-urban area (Table 2). HIV-1 prevalence was higher in this sentinel group than in most age groups in the general population, but differences in prevalence varied considerably between age groups (Fig. 1). This sentinel group comprised mainly women; rural women were over-represented.

Only 33 patients (all urban) with suspected STD were screened for syphilis serology at the STD clinic during the study. Eleven (33%) were HIV-1 seropositive. STD patients (approximately equal numbers of men and women) screened for syphilis had the highest standardized prevalence ratio of all urban sentinel groups (Table 2).

The crude HIV-1 prevalence in antenatal clinic attenders was 12% (138 out of 1193). The standardized HIV-1 prevalence in this group was 25% lower [95% confidence interval (CI), 2–42] than that in urban women aged 15–44 years in the population survey (Table 2). Most antenatal clinic attenders were less than 35 years old. Although HIV-1 prevalence in urban women in the general population in was much lower in those aged 35 years and above than in those aged less than 35 years, this was not reflected in antenatal clinic attenders (Fig. 1).

Discussion

At present, blood donors who are related to blood recipients appear to be a representative group for HIV-1 serosurveillance in Mwanza Region, provided data are standardized by age, sex, and urban/non-urban location. Standardization for hospital location is important because more blood transfusions take place in urban areas, where HIV-1 prevalence is higher.

Using blood donors as a sentinel group requires HIV-1 testing with a high sensitivity and specificity in district hospitals, as well as accurate recording and processing of data. The zonal referral hospital (Bugando Medical Centre) had performed monthly quality control of test performance in district (and other) hospitals it supervises in the region for 1.5 years. The errors detected in data entry at national level had little impact on the observed HIV-1 prevalence.

Outpatients examined for malaria or anaemia had higher HIV-1 prevalence than the general population, particularly in the non-urban area, probably because of selection bias. Four of the five non-urban district hospitals are in roadside settlements. People living near the hospital are likely to be over-represented among outpatients [13], particularly for complaints such as fever, for which there are many alternative treatment sites (for example, dispensaries and shops). Alternatively, the high HIV-1 prevalence among patients examined for malaria could be due to the higher frequency of fever in HIV-1 infected people (due to causes other than malaria) [14]. If these biases do not vary greatly over time, these two groups of outpatients could be used as sentinel groups in which follow trends. Women aged 15–34 years constituted 79% of patients examined for anaemia. Because patients examined for the presence of malaria parasites were more evenly distributed over the age, sex and residence groups, they provide a more precise estimate of HIV-1 prevalence in the various subgroups.

As expected, patients reporting STD who were screened for syphilis had a markedly increased HIV-1 prevalence [15]. However, relatively few such patients presented themselves, and so estimates for this group are of limited precision. Use of another screening technique (for example, on saliva) could increase the STD patient sample size.

Surprisingly, the HIV-1 prevalence in antenatal clinic attenders was significantly lower than that of women in the general population. The distribution of HIV-1 prevalence by age was also different in antenatal clinic attenders than in the general population. Young women at high risk of HIV-1 infection may have lower fertility rates, because of contraceptive use or STD-induced infertility. Alternatively, women in this group may have attended antenatal clinics elsewhere (for example, in the private sector) or not have received antenatal care at all. Although antenatal clinic attenders were not as representative as might have been expected [2], they might be a suitable group to monitor trends, provided the selection bias does not vary much over time.

Criteria other than representativeness are also important for judging the suitability of groups for sentinel surveillance. These include accessibility, ease of maintaining confidentiality and cost [1-3]. The accessibility of all sentinel groups in this study was good, since they were all hospital attenders having blood taken for purposes other than HIV-1 testing. HIV-1 testing was unlinked in all sentinel groups and, except in blood donors, all blood was taken for reasons other than HIV-1 testing, facilitating confidentiality. Unlinked testing also minimizes participation bias. [1,2,16,17]

Because resources available for AIDS control are limited, the cost of sentinel surveillance has to be kept to a minimum; the majority of resources should be spent on interventions to reduce HIV-1 transmission. Pregnant women could be a suitable sentinel group, because HIV-1 infection in pregnant women has immediate consequences for the health of mothers and children. However, at present most Tanzanian antenatal clinics do not routinely screen for syphilis or anaemia, and can therefore provide only limited sentinel surveillance. These screening services could be expanded, but at a cost. Because blood donors have to be tested for HIV-1 to prevent transmission through blood transfusions, using this group for sentinel surveillance has the great advantage that no extra tests are required.

Using filter paper to collect, transport and store samples of capillary blood proved to be very convenient. The method was easily introduced, allowed blood samples to be collected in laboratories where venous blood is rarely drawn, and did not require refrigerators for storage or coolboxes for transport, enabling all samples to be tested in the referral hospital, using the same test kits. The main problem was that insufficient blood was collected on the filter paper in some sites. However, this proved fairly easy to correct by supervisory visits, if detected in time. Therefore, for sentinel groups other than blood donors, the filter paper method for the collection, transport and storage of blood samples is highly recommended.

We conclude that at present blood donors who are related to blood recipients are a representative sentinel group in Mwanza Region, provided that prevalence rates are standardised for age, sex, and hospital location. This group is also the least costly to follow for sentinel surveillance. Like the other sentinel groups discussed in this paper, blood donors are easily accessible and confidentiality can easily be maintained. However, self-selection of blood donors may increase, particularly if linked testing and counselling become more widely available. Therefore, the representativeness of various sentinel groups over time should be assessed whenever a population survey is carried out. If this assessment is repeated in an area, it might also show whether trends are accurately reflected by antenatal clinic attenders or patients with fever.

Acknowledgements

We thank the Principal Secretary, Ministry of Health, and the Director-General of the National Institute for Medical Research, Dar es Salaam, Tanzania, for permission to carry out and publish the results of this study. We are grateful to the district medical officers, medical officers-in-charge, and laboratory staff of the (designated) district hospitals for their support.

Sponsorship: Supported by Netherlands Minister for Development Co-operation (Department DST/SO) as part of the Tanzania-Netherlands Research Project on AIDS and HIV Infection (TANERA). Salary support was received from the Wellcome Trust (A.N.) and the Overseas Development Administration (A.N. and H.G.)

References

1. Chin J: Public health surveillance of AIDS and HIV infections. Bulletin of the World Health Organization 1990, 68:529-536.
2. Slutkin G, Chin J, Tarantola D, Mann J: Sentinel surveillance for HIV infection - A method to monitor HIV infection trends in population groups. Geneva: World Health Organization/Global Programme on AIDS, 1988.
3. Global Programme on AIDS: Field guidelines for HIV sentinel surveillance - A manual for national AIDS control programmes. Geneva: World Health Organization, 1989.
4. Klokke AH, Kigadye FC, Schalula PJJ: Evaluation of HIV testing of blood-spotted paper samples [letter]. Tropical Doctor 1991,21:120.
5. Farzadegan H, Quinn T, Polk BF: Detecting antibodies to human immunodeficiency virus in dried blood on filter papers [letter]. J Infect Dis 1987,155:1073-1074.
6. Van den Akker R, Kooy H, Van der Meyden HP, Lumey BH: Recovery of HIV antibodies in eluates from plasma and erythrocytes dried on filter paper and stored under various conditions [letter]. AIDS 1990, 4:90-91.
7. Hoff R, Berardi VP, Weiblen BJ, Mahoney-Trout L, Mitchell ML, Grady GF: Seroprevalence of human immunodeficiency virus among childbearing women - estimation by testing samples of blood from newborns. New Engl J Med 1988, 318:525-530.
8. Novick LF, Berns D, Stricof R, Stevens R, Pass K, Wethers J: HIV seroprevalence in newborns in New York State. JAMA 1989, 261:1745-1750.
9. Peckham CS, Tedder RS, Briggs M, et al: Prevalence of maternal HIV infection based on unlinked anonymous testing of newborn babies. Lancet 1990, 335:516-519.
10. Ippolito G, Costa F, Stegagno M, Angeloni P, Angeloni U, Guzzanti E: Blind serosurvey of HIV antibodies in newborns in 92 Italian hospitals: a method for monitoring the infection rate in women at time of delivery. J Acquir Immune Defic Syndr. 1991, 4:402-407.
11. Barongo LR, Borgdorff MW, Mosha FF, et al: The epidemiology of HIV-1 infection in urban areas, roadside settlements and rural villages in Mwanza Region, Tanzania. AIDS 1992, 6:1521-1528.
12. Breslow NE, Day NE: Statistical methods in cancer research. Volume II. The design and analysis of cohort studies. Lyon: International Agency for Research on Cancer (IARC), 1987.
13. Stock R: Distances and the utilization of health facilities in rural Nigeria. Social Science and Medicine 1983, 17:563-570.

14. Greenberg AE, Nsa W, Ryder RW, et al: Plasmodium falciparum malaria and perinatally acquired human immunodeficiency virus type 1 infection in Kinshasa, Zaire - a prospective longitudinal cohort study of 587 children. New Engl J Med 1991, 325:105-109.

15. Piot P, Plummer FA, Mhalu FS, Lamboray JL, Chin J, Mann JM: AIDS: an international perspective. Science 1988, 239:573-579.

16. Hull HF, Bettinger CJ, Gallaher MM, Keller NM, Wilson J, Mertz GJ: Comparison of HIV-antibody prevalence in patients consenting to and declining HIV-antibody testing in an STD clinic. JAMA 1988, 260:935-938.

17. Barbacci M, Repke JT, Chaisson RE: Routine prenatal screening for HIV infection. Lancet 1991, 337:709-711.

5

HIV-1 infection as a risk factor for the development of tuberculosis: a case-control study in Tanzania

J. van den Broek[1], MW Borgdorff[2,4], NG Pakker[5], HJ Chum[1],AH Klokke[3], KP Senkoro[2] and JN Newell[6,7]

International Journal of Epidemiology 1993; 22: 1159-1165

Summary

A population based case-control study was carried out in Mwanza Region, Tanzania, to determine the relative and population attributable risk of human immunodeficiency virus type 1 (HIV-1) infection for developing active tuberculosis. Cases were 441 consecutively diagnosed patients with tuberculosis (all types), aged 15–54 years. Controls were a representative population sample of 4,161 people, drawn in a stratified cluster sample from urban areas, roadside settlements, and rural villages. HIV-1 infection was determined by ELISA and if the ELISA result was indeterminate by Western Blot.

The HIV-1 prevalence in cases was 23.0% in rural, 32.1% in roadside, and 54.1% in urban areas, while in controls these prevalences were 3.4%, 7.2% and 12.1% respectively. The relative risk (RR) of HIV-1 infection for the development of active tuberculosis was estimated to be 8.3 (95% confidence interval [CI] 6.4–11.0). This risk varied little by sex or residence, but appeared to be more pronounced in the age group 25–34 years. The case detection rate of tuberculosis in those aged 15–54 years was 125/100,000 people per year. The population attributable risk was 36/100,000 persons per year, implying that 29% of tuberculosis cases at present may be attributable to HIV-1 infection. It is concluded that HIV-1 infection is a major contributing factor to the increased case detection rate of tuberculosis observed over the past 10 years in Mwanza Region. If the prevalence of HIV-1 continues to increase, the incidence of tuberculosis will continue to rise as well. Maintaining a high cure rate of tuberculosis patients will be imperative to prevent an increased risk of tuberculosis infection to HIV-1 infected and uninfected people.

1 National Tuberculosis/Leprosy Programme, Dar es Salaam, Tanzania
2 National Institute for Medical Research, Mwanza, Tanzania
3 Bugando Medical Centre, Mwanza, Tanzania
4 Royal Tropical Institute, Amsterdam, The Netherlands
5 Nijmegen Institute for International Health, Nijmegen, The Netherlands
6 African Medical and Research Foundation, Mwanza, Tanzania
7 London School of Hygiene and Tropical Medicine, London, UK

Introduction

In recent years the case detection rate of tuberculosis has increased in a number of countries in East Africa, for instance in Malawi [1] and Tanzania [2], and also in the USA. [3] This increase is recent, as up to 10 years ago the incidence of tuberculosis infection and active tuberculosis was steeply declining in many countries, and slowly declining or remaining stable in much of Africa. [4] Human immunodeficiency virus type 1 (HIV-1) infection is thought to be an important contributing factor to this recent increase. In hospital-based case-control studies in Haiti [5] and Ivory Coast [6] and a population based case-control study in Malawi [7] a strong association was shown between HIV-1 infection and active tuberculosis. In a cohort of women in Zaire the risk of tuberculosis in HIV-1 infected women was 26 times that in non HIV-1 infected women [8] and in the USA the incidence of tuberculosis was significantly higher in HIV-1 positive intravenous drugs users than in HIV-1 negative controls. [9]

In Mwanza Region the case detection rate of tuberculosis (all forms) has increased by 47% from 64/100,000 in 1982 to 94/100,000 in 1991 (Figure 1) giving an annual increase of 4% over the past 10 years. From 1982 the proportion of cases which were smear-negative or extra-pulmonary increased from 20% to 39%.

Mwanza Region is situated on the shores of Lake Victoria in north-west Tanzania, and has a population of 2 million. In this Region two studies were carried out almost simultaneously: HIV-1 testing of tuberculosis patients by the National Tuberculosis/ Leprosy Programme, as part of a collaborative study of the International Union Against Tuberculosis and Lung Disease, the World Health Organisation and the Tanzania National Tuberculosis and Leprosy Programme (April–September 1991); and a popula-

Figure 1. The case detection rates of tuberculosis in Mwanza Region from 1978 to 1991

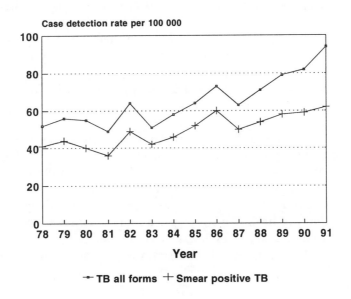

tion survey by the National Institute for Medical Research, as part of the Tanzania-Netherlands Research Project on AIDS and HIV-1 Infection, and the STD/HIV Intervention Project (August 1990–February 1991). This provided the opportunity for a population based case-control study to determine the relative and population attributable risk of HIV-1 infection for developing active tuberculosis.

Methods

Cases

From April to September 1991 all newly diagnosed cases of pulmonary and extra-pulmonary tuberculosis, aged 15–54 years and resident in Mwanza Region, who were started on anti-tuberculosis treatment, were enroled in the study. Included were relapsed cases who had been declared cured in the past. Excluded were patients who had started treatment elsewhere and were transferred while on treatment, and patients returning to treatment after defaulting. The intake took place in all nine hospitals of Mwanza region.

Information was recorded on sex, age and residence. All patients were clinically examined, and had at least two sputum smears taken. Sputum smears were examined locally by Ziehl-Neelsen staining and direct microscopy. A second sputum smear was sent to Bugando Medical Centre, the reference laboratory, where the smears were stained with auramin and examined by fluorescence microscopy. Sputum was also cultured, and positive specimens were sent to the central tuberculosis laboratory of Muhimbili Medical Centre in Dar es Salaam for repeat culture and sensitivity testing. Although not all hospitals had x-ray facilities 289/441 (66%) of the cases had a chest x-ray taken which was examined by at least one medical doctor.

The definitions we used in this study were:
- Smear-positive pulmonary tuberculosis: patient with a positive smear in the reference laboratory; or with a positive local smear confirmed by a positive culture.
- Smear-negative pulmonary tuberculosis: patient with clinical evidence of pulmonary tuberculosis, diagnosed by a medical doctor, an abnormal chest x-ray and no positive sputum smear.
- Extra-pulmonary tuberculosis: patient with clinical evidence of extra-pulmonary tuberculosis, diagnosed by a medical doctor.

A 5–10 ml sample of venous blood was collected from all cases, as soon as possible after starting treatment for tuberculosis. HIV-1 antibodies were demonstrated by ELISA (Vironostika anti-HTLV-III, Organon Teknika, The Netherlands). On all samples with indeterminate results and on a further random sample of 54, Western Blot was performed (Novopath, Bio-rad, Hercules, California) showing a sensitivity of 97% (23/24) and a specificity of 100% (29/29) compared with Western Blot (the one Western Blot with an indeterminate result was excluded from these calculations). The negative predictive value of ELISA was 96%, the positive predictive value 100%.

Controls

A full report on the population survey has been published elsewhere. [10] For the selection of controls, Mwanza Region was divided into three strata: urban, roadside and rural. The urban stratum comprised Mwanza Municipality; the roadside stratum was made up of the small towns and villages along the main roads; and the rural stratum consisted of all other villages. From each stratum, 20 sites were randomly selected, with the probability of selection proportional to population size. Within selected sites, 10-cell units were selected using simple random sampling to give an average total of 100 eligible individuals, aged 15–54 years, in each rural site and 50 eligible individuals in each roadside and urban site. (A 10-cell unit comprises 10 households.) Because of variability in the sizes of 10-cell units, the final numbers selected for inclusion in the rural, roadside and urban strata were 2,434, 1,157, and 1,554 respectively. The number of individuals giving a blood sample in the three strata were 2,019, 958 and 1,184 respectively, equivalent to response rates of 83%, 83%, and 76%. Variables recorded included age, sex, and residence. A 5–10 ml sample of venous blood was taken and separated in the field. The fieldwork took place from August 1990 to February 1991. Serum was tested for HIV-1 antibodies with ELISA (Vironostika anti-HTLV-III, Organon Teknika, The Netherlands). All 268 positive samples underwent confirmatory testing using Western Blot (Organon, Epitope Inc, USA). To ensure comparability of HIV-1 test results between cases and controls, ELISA results have been used for all samples to determine HIV-1 infection except for an indeterminate ELISA where we used the Western Blot result.

Data analysis

Cases and controls were subdivided by residential strata, sex, and age group. Exact Mantel-Haenszel odds ratios (OR) were calculated with the EGRET program to summarize over subgroups and have been used as estimates of relative risk.

As HIV-1 infection was not associated with type of tuberculosis in this study, all cases of tuberculosis have been taken together for calculation of the OR.

In order to calculate the case detection rate and population attributable risk the following were calculated. The number of cases by age, sex and residence identified in the various hospitals was multiplied by 365 divided by the intake time in days in order to obtain an estimate of the annual number of cases detected, separately for HIV-1 positive and HIV-1 negative cases. From data of the 1978 and 1988 censuses, an extrapolation was made to estimate the population of Mwanza Region in 1991 by age, sex, and residence. By applying the HIV-1 prevalence rates found in the population survey the numbers of HIV-1 positive and HIV-1 negative individuals in the population were estimated. The population attributable risk was calculated as: (case detection rate of tuberculosis in total population) - (case detection rate of tuberculosis in HIV-1 uninfected).

The quarterly numbers of cases of smear-positive tuberculosis detected in those aged 15–54 years were retrieved from the routine information system from 1989 to 1992. Regression analysis was used to estimate the expected number of cases in each quarter. The ratio of the observed and expected number of cases in the second and third quarter of 1991 was used to estimate the magnitude of the bias caused by calculating annual rates from cases collected in only part of the year.

Results

In the study period 441 cases of tuberculosis were identified, according to the definitions and exclusion criteria adopted for this study. The distribution of age, sex and residence of cases and controls is presented in Table 1. Tuberculosis patients were on average older than controls ($z=6.57$, $P<0.0001$) and a higher proportion of them were males ($\chi^2=32.0$, $P<0.0001$). Due to the sampling scheme adopted for controls, the residence of tuberculosis patients was more often the rural villages ($\chi^2=38.4$, $P<0.0001$).

The prevalence of HIV-1 infection among various categories of tuberculosis patients is shown in Table 2. There is no statistically significant association between HIV-1 infection and the type of tuberculosis ($\chi^2= 0.82$, df 3, $P>0.05$).

The prevalence of HIV-1 infection in cases and controls by age, sex, and residence is presented in Table 3. HIV-1 prevalence was much higher in cases than in controls for most subgroups. The HIV-1 prevalence in cases was 23.0% in rural, 32.1% in roadside, and 54.1% in urban areas, while in controls these prevalences were 3.4%, 7.2% and 12.1% respectively.

Table 1.   Age, sex and residence of tuberculosis cases and population controls

		Tuberculosis cases		Population controls	
		No.	(%)	No.	(%)
Sex	Male	275	(62.4)	2000	(48.1)
	Female	166	(37.6)	2161	(51.9)
Age (years)	15-24	88	(20.0)	1495	(35.9)
	25-34	169	(38.3)	1385	(33.3)
	35-44	103	(23.4)	770	(18.5)
	45-54	81	(18.4)	511	(12.3)
Residence	Rural	283	(64.2)	2019	(48.5)
	Roadside	84	(19.0)	958	(23.0)
	Urban	74	(16.8)	1184	(28.5)
Total		441	(100)	4161	(100)

Table 2.   HIV-1 prevalence in patients with various types of tuberculosis disease

Type of tuberculosis	HIV-1 + ve		Total (100%)
	No.	(%)	
Smear positive	110	(30.4)	362
Relapses	5	(23.8)	21
Smear negative	13	(31.7)	41
Extra-pulmonary	4	(23.5)	17
Total	132	(29.9)	441

Table 3. HIV-1 prevalence in cases and controls by age, sex, and residence

Age group (years)	Cases No.	(%)	Controls No.	(%)	Cases No.	(%)	Controls No.	(%)
		Male				Female		
			Rural					
15-24	5/24	(21)	5/314	(1.6)	3/23	(13)	17/397	(4.3)
25-34	26/65	(40)	12/309	(3.9)	15/45	(33)	10/330	(3.0)
35-44	9/45	(20)	6/191	(3.1)	6/23	(26)	9/210	(4.3)
45-54	0/45	(0)	6/160	(3.8)	1/13	(8)	3/108	(2.8)
Subtotal	40/179	(22)	29/974	(3.0)	25/104	(24)	39/1045	(3.7)
			Roadside					
15-24	1/8	(13)	2/134	(1.5)	4/13	(31)	18/183	(9.8)
25-34	5/15	(33)	12/142	(8.5)	8/15	(53)	20/193	(10.4)
35-44	4/15	(27)	9/84	(10.7)	2/6	(33)	5/83	(6.0)
45-54	2/6	(33)	2/71	(2.8)	1/6	(17)	1/68	(1.5)
Subtotal	12/44	(27)	25/431	(5.8)	15/40	(38)	44/527	(8.3)
			Urban					
15-24	5/14	(36)	14/222	(6.3)	2/6	(33)	38/245	(15.5)
25-34	13/19	(68)	21/198	(10.6)	8/10	(80)	41/213	(19.2)
35-44	6/9	(67)	15/116	(12.9)	3/5	(60)	8/86	(9.3)
45-54	3/10	(30)	4/59	(6.8)	0/1	(0)	2/45	(4.4)
Subtotal	27/52	(52)	54/595	(9.1)	13/22	(59)	89/589	(15.1)
Total	79/275	(29)	108/2000	(5.4)	53/166	(32)	172/2161	(8.0)

The OR that can be calculated from Table 3 are presented in Table 4. The overall Mantel Haenszel OR is 8.3 (95% confidence interval (CI): 6.4–11.0). The Mantel Haenszel OR for the two sexes and the three residential strata are similar. The OR appeared to be highest in those aged 25–34 years and lowest in those aged 45–54 years.

The case detection rate in the age group 15–54 years was 125/100,000 per year. The population attributable risk was 36/100,000 per year. If the association between HIV-1 infection and tuberculosis were causal, 29% of tuberculosis cases occurring at present would be attributable to HIV-1 infection.

The quarterly numbers of cases of smear-positive tuberculosis detected in those aged 15–54 years from 1989 to 1992 are shown in Figure 2. The quarterly variation in the numbers of cases detected does not show a seasonal pattern. Using linear regression the expected number of cases in the second and third quarter of 1991 was calculated to be 269 + 275 = 544, while the observed number was 252 + 223 = 475, giving a ratio of observed/expected number of cases of 0.87.

Table 4. Relative risks of HIV-1 infection for the development of tuberculosis disease

		Odds ratio	95% confidence interval
Sex	Male	8.9	6.1 - 12.9
	Female	7.7	5.1 - 11.7
Age (years)	15-24	5.7	3.1 - 10.4
	25-34	13.4	8.8 - 20.7
	35-44	7.3	4.1 - 13.2
	45-54	2.9	1.0 - 7.9
Residence	Rural	8.8	5.9 - 13.1
	Roadside	6.1	3.4 - 10.7
	Urban	10.2	5.9 - 17.9
Total		8.3	6.4 - 11.0

Figure 2. Number of smear-positive tuberculosis cases aged 15-54 yeaars, diagnosed in Mwanza Region by quarter, 1989-1992

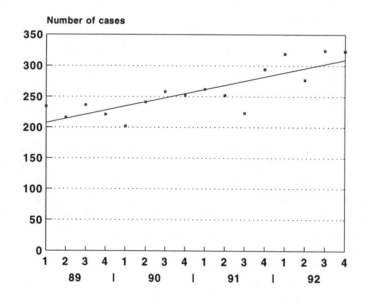

Discussion

This population-based study shows a strong association between HIV-1 infection and the development of active tuberculosis, with a relative risk (estimated by the OR) of 8.3, implying that HIV-1 infected individuals are 8.3 times more likely to develop tuberculosis than those who are not infected with HIV-1. While the population attributable risk is high at 36/100,000 per year – it is higher than the total incidence of tuberculosis in many countries – it may be expected to rise further if the prevalence of HIV-1 infection continues to increase. It is likely that at present 29% of tuberculosis cases in Mwanza Region occur as a consequence of HIV-1 infection.

Some controls may have been suffering from active tuberculosis, as during the population survey no screening for tuberculosis took place. However, because of the low population prevalence of tuberculosis disease, this number is likely to be small: with an incidence of 125/100,000 per year and a mean duration of active tuberculosis of less than four years, the prevalence of disease would be $< 500/100,000$ i.e. $< 0.5\%$. Exclusion of cases in the control group would theoretically lead to a higher estimate of the OR, but in the present study this effect would have been very small.

The quarterly variation in the numbers of cases of smear-positive tuberculosis detected in those aged 15–54 years does not show a seasonal pattern. However, in the study period the number of smear-positive cases detected was 87% of the number of cases expected. Quarterly variation in the numbers of cases of smear-negative tuberculosis is difficult to assess, because the case definition for smear-negative tuberculosis used by the services is less strict than the one applied in this study. As a large majority of cases diagnosed with tuberculosis in this Region is smear-positive (82% in this study) trends in the number of newly detected smear-positive cases should be closely associated with, although not be identical to trends in total numbers of tuberculosis cases. Therefore, it may be argued that a better estimate of the annual case detection rate and population attributable risk would be obtained by multiplying the results presented above by 1.15 (1/0.87) giving 144 and 45 per 100,000 respectively.

It is possible that tuberculosis cases in more urbanized settings find their way to the health care service more easily than those in remote places. Because HIV-1 prevalence is higher in urban settings, this selection bias would lead to an overestimate of the OR. We do not believe selection bias has been a major influence on our results, because the residence of cases has been classified according to where the patients lived rather than where they were diagnosed, and because the OR is the same for all three residential strata.

The high relative risk of HIV-1 infection for the development of active tuberculosis has also been shown by studies in Haiti [5], Ivory Coast [6], Malawi [7] and Zaire. [8] In Ivory Coast the OR associated with HIV-1 was 4.7 (95% CI: 3.6–6.2). In Haiti the OR associated with HIV-1 infection were shown to be 15.7 (95% CI: 4.8–50.0) for the age group 20–39, and 3.0 (95% CI: 0.8–11.1) for those aged 40-59 years. In Zaire the relative risk was found to be 26 (95% CI: 5–125) for all forms of tuberculosis and 10 (95% CI: 1.5–47) for bacteriologically-confirmed pulmonary tuberculosis. In the population-based study in Malawi the OR was 7.4 (95% CI: 3.3–16.7).

In the present study, the OR appears to be highest in the age group 25–34 years and lowest in the age group 45–54 years, which is consistent with the findings in Haiti. It is unclear why young adults would have excess risk of developing tuberculosis when they are HIV-1 infected, compared to other age groups. HIV-1 infection greatly increases the risk of active tuberculosis in those who have been newly infected with tuberculosis bacilli. [11,12] If HIV-1 infection is a stronger risk factor for the development of tuberculosis in those newly infected with tuberculosis than in those previously infected (who develop the disease by reactivation) and if the incidence of new tuberculosis infections were higher in young adults than in older ones, this might result in a higher OR.

Ten years ago the case detection rate of tuberculosis was 32% below the current level. Of the tuberculosis cases detected at present 29% is attributable to HIV-1 infection. It may be concluded that HIV-1 infection has contributed substantially to an increased incidence of tuberculosis in Mwanza Region. Unless the cure rate of tuberculosis patients is maintained at a high level or even improved, the increased incidence of tuberculosis – in particular smear-positive tuberculosis – is likely to lead to an increased risk of tuberculosis infection to both HIV-1 infected and uninfected people.

Acknowledgements

We thank the Principal Secretary, Ministry of Health, and the Director-General of the National Institute for Medical Research for permission to carry out and publish the results of this study. We are grateful to the district medical officers, the district tuberculosis and leprosy co-ordinators, and laboratory staff of the hospitals in Mwanza Region for their support. Special thanks are due to Mr Mugomela, of the reference tuberculosis laboratory of Bugando Medical Centre, and Mr Chonde, of the reference tuberculosis laboratory of Muhimbili Medical Centre. Data collection on tuberculosis cases was financed by the International Union Against Tuberculosis and Lung Diseases and the World Health Organisation and the population survey by the Netherlands Minister for Development Co-operation and the AIDS Task Force of the European Community. We thank Prof R A Coutinho for critically reviewing the manuscript.

References

1. Styblo K. Impact of HIV infection on the global epidemiology of tuberculosis. Bull Int Union Tuberc Lung Dis, 1991; 66:27-32.
2. Chum HJ. Ten years of the National Tuberculosis/Leprosy Programme in Tanzania. Bull Int Union Tuberc Lung Dis 1989; 64:34-36.
3. Rieder HL, Cauthen GM, Kelly GD, Bloch AB, Snider DE, Tuberculosis in the United States. JAMA, 1989;262:385-389.
4. Styblo K, Enarson DA, Epidemiology of tuberculosis. Selected papers No 24, The Hague: KNCV 1991.
5. Long R, Scalcini M, Manfreda J, et al. Impact of human immunodeficiency virus type I on tuberculosis in rural Haiti. Am Rev Respir Dis 1991; 143:69-73.

6. Cock KM De, Gnaore E, Adjorlolo G, et al. Risk of tuberculosis in patients with HIV-1 and HIV-2 infections in Abidjan, Ivory Coast. BMJ 1991;302:496-499.

7. Ponnighaus JM, Mwanjasi LJ, Fine PEM, et al. Is HIV infection a risk factor for leprosy? Int J Lepr 1991;59:221-228.

8. Braun MM, Badi N, Ryder RW, et al. A retrospective cohort study of the risk of tuberculosis among women of childbearing age with HIV infection in Zaire. Am Rev Respir Dis 1991;143:501-504.

9. Selwyn PA, Hartel D, Lewis VA, et al. A prospective study of the risk of tuberculosis among intravenous drug users with human immunodeficiency virus infection. New Eng J Med 1989;320:45-350.

10. Barongo LR, Borgdorff MW, Mosha FF, et al. The epidemiology of HIV-1 infection in urban areas, roadside settlements and rural villages in Mwanza Region, Tanzania. AIDS 1992;6:1521-1528.

11. Daley CL, Small PM, Schecter GF, et al. An outbreak of tuberculosis with accelerated progression among persons infected with the human immunodeficiency virus. N Eng J Med 1991;326:231-235.

12. Perri, G Di, Cruciani M, Danzi MC, et al. Nosocomial epidemic of active tuberculosis among HIV-infected. Lancet; 1989:1502-1504.

6

HIV-1 infection as a risk factor for leprosy:

a case-control study in Tanzania

Martien W Borgdorff, MD [1,4], *Jacques van den Broek, MD* [2], *Hamsa J Chum, MD* [2], *Arnoud H Klokke, MSc* [3], *Petra Graf, MD* [2], *Longin R Barongo, MD* [1], *James N Newell, PhD* [5,6]

International Journal of Leprosy 1993; 61: 556-562*

Summary

A case-control study was carried out in Tanzania to determine the relative risk of those with
HIV-1 infection for getting leprosy. Cases were 93 consecutively diagnosed patients with leprosy
aged 15–54 years from the Mwanza Region. Controls were a representative population sample
of 4161 people drawn from a stratified cluster sample from urban areas, roadside settlements,
and rural villages. HIV-1 infection was determined by enzyme-linked immunosorbent assay
(ELISA); Western blot was used when the ELISA result was indeterminate.

The HIV-1 prevalence in leprosy cases was 10% in rural (7 of 72) and in roadside and urban
areas (2 of 21); in controls these prevalences were 3.4% and 9.9%, respectively. The relative
risk of HIV-1 infection for the development of leprosy was estimated to be 2.2 [95% confidence
interval (CI) = 1.0–4.7; p=0.07]. HIV-1 infection was significantly associated with multibacillary
(MB) leprosy (odds ratio 4.6; CI = 1.3–13.2) but not with paucibacillary leprosy (odds ratio 1.4;
95% CI = 0.4–3.8). The population etiological fraction for the development of MB leprosy
attributable to HIV-1 infection in this population is estimated to be 13% (95% CI = 4%–23%). We
conclude that HIV-1 is a risk factor for the development of MB leprosy. The impact of the HIV-1
epidemic on the incidence of leprosy so far has been limited since HIV-1 occurs mainly in urban
areas and leprosy in rural areas.

1 National Institute for Medical Research, Mwanza, Tanzania
2 National Tuberculosis/Leprosy Programme, Dar es Salaam, Tanzania
3 Bugando Medical Centre, Mwanza, Tanzania
4 Royal Tropical Institute, Amsterdam, The Netherlands
5 African Medical and Research Foundation, Mwanza, Tanzania
6 London School of Hygiene and Tropical Medicine, London, UK

* Received for publication

Introduction

Although HIV-1 infection has been shown to be strongly associated with the development of active tuberculosis [4,5,10,16] and disease caused by other mycobacteria [1,12], its association with leprosy is much less clear. In a hospital-based case-control study in Zambia [11] an association was shown between HIV-1 infection and leprosy, but this was not confirmed in other hospital-based studies in Ethiopia [17] and Yemen and various countries in Africa [8] nor in a community-based study in Malawi [13].

The Mwanza Region is situated on the shores of Lake Victoria in north-west Tanzania, and has a population of two million. In this region two studies were carried out around the same time: HIV-1 testing of leprosy and tuberculosis patients by the National Tuberculosis/Leprosy Program, as part of a collaborative study of the International Union Against Tuberculosis and Lung Disease, the World Health Organization, and the Tanzania National Tuberculosis and Leprosy Program (April–September 1991); and a population survey by the National Institute for Medical Research, as part of the Tanzania-Netherlands Research Project on AIDS and HIV Infection, and AMREF's STD/HIV Intervention Project (August 1990–February 1991). This provided the opportunity for a secondary data analysis in which data on leprosy cases were combined with data on population controls in a case-control study to determine the relative risk of HIV-1 infection for developing leprosy. A similar comparison between tuberculosis cases and population controls is reported separately [18].

Methods

Cases
From April to September 1991 all 93 newly diagnosed cases of leprosy, aged 15–54 years from the Mwanza Region who were started on treatment, were enrolled in the study. Included were seven relapsed cases who had been declared cured in the past. Excluded were patients who had started treatment elsewhere and were transferred in while on treatment, patients not resident in the Mwanza Region, and patients returning to treatment after defaulting. The intake took place in all nine hospitals of the Mwanza Region.

Information was recorded on sex, age and residence. All patients were examined clinically by experienced field supervisors. The standard clinical examination forms were all scrutinized by an experienced Medical Officer (JvdB), who also examined all cases with an unclear classification. The Ridley-Jopling classification was used [6], with the modification that midborderline (BB) leprosy was classified as either borderline lepromatous (BL) or borderline tuberculoid (BT) leprosy. From each patient four slit-skin smears were taken. The skin smears were examined locally and in the reference laboratory (Bugando Medical Center) by Ziehl-Neelsen staining and direct microscopy. Results were graded negative if no *Mycobacterium leprae* were seen in 100 fields, and positive if the bacterial index (BI) was 1+ or more on the Ridley logarithmic scale [14,19], i.e., if at least one bacillus was detected in 100 fields examined. Skin biopsies were not taken routinely. Clinical and microbiological classification of leprosy cases occurred blind to HIV-1 status.

The definitions used in this study were [19,20,21]: a) Multibacillary leprosy: a clinical presentation consistent with lepromatous (LL) or borderline lepromatous (BL) leprosy or at least one skin smear with a BI of 1 + or more. b) Paucibacillary leprosy: a clinical presentation of tuberculoid (TT) or borderline tuberculoid (BT) leprosy and a BI of 0.

A 5–10 ml sample of venous blood was collected from all cases as soon as possible after starting treatment for leprosy. HIV-1 antibodies were demonstrated by ELISA (Vironostika anti-HTLV-III; Organon Teknika, Boxtel, The Netherlands). On all samples with indeterminate ELISA results Western Blot was performed (Novopath; Bio-rad, Hercules, California, USA).

Controls
A full report on the population survey, which was carried out from August 1990 to February 1991, has been published elsewhere [2]. For the selection of controls, the Mwanza Region was divided into three strata: urban, roadside and rural. The urban stratum comprised Mwanza Municipality; the roadside stratum was made up of the small towns and villages along the main roads; and the rural stratum consisted of all other villages. From each stratum, 20 sites were randomly selected, with the probability of selection proportional to population size. Within selected sites, ten-cell units were selected using a simple random sampling to give an average total of 100 eligible individuals, aged 15–54 years, in each rural site and 50 eligible individuals in each roadside and urban site. (A ten-cell unit comprises on average ten households.) Because of variability in the sizes of the ten-cell units, the final numbers selected for inclusion in the rural, roadside and urban strata were 2434, 1157, and 1554, respectively. The number of study participants in the three strata were 2019, 958, and 1184, giving participation rates of 83%, 83%, and 76%, respectively. Variables recorded included age, sex, and residence. Venous blood (5–10 ml) was taken and separated in the field. Serum was tested for HIV-1 antibodies with ELISA (Organon Teknika). All non-negative samples underwent confirmatory testing using Western Blot (Organon; Epitope, Beaverton, Oregon, USA).

Data analysis
Cases and controls were subdivided by residential strata, sex, and age groups. Due to the small number of leprosy cases in the urban and roadside strata, these strata were combined in the analysis. In order to make the HIV-1 results between cases and controls comparable, HIV-1 status in both groups was based on the ELISA results; for those with an indeterminate ELISA result the Western blot result was used. The Western blot was considered positive if at least two of the gp41, gp120, and gp160 bands were present [22]. Odds ratios (ORs) and their confidence intervals were calculated with the exact method (EGRET computer program), summarizing over subgroups after stratification by age, sex, and residence, and are used as estimates of relative risk. The population etiological fraction was estimated taking into account stratification of the sample by residence, age, and sex using the following formula [15]:

$$\lambda = \Sigma\, n_i\, \lambda_i \,/\, \Sigma\, n_i$$

where λ is the population etiological fraction, n_i is the number of cases in stratum i, and λ_i is the etiological fraction for stratum i. λ_i is calculated as:

$$\lambda_i = (a_i d_i - b_i c_i)/(n_i d_i)$$

where a_i is the number of exposed cases, d_i the number of unexposed controls, b_i the number of exposed controls, c_i the number of unexposed cases, and n_i the number of cases in stratum i. Strata with 0 cases were ignored. The variance and confidence intervals were also calculated according to Schlesselmann [15].

Results

In the study period 93 cases of leprosy were identified. The distribution of age, sex and residence of cases and controls is presented in Table 1. Leprosy patients were, on the average, older than controls and a higher proportion of them were males. The residence of the leprosy patients was more often the rural villages. The geographic distribution of the leprosy cases identified in this study is presented in Figure 1.

Of the 93 cases, 28 had multibacillary (MB) leprosy (LL 10, BL 18), and 65 had paucibacillary (PB) leprosy (BT 44, TT 21). All LL and 16 out of 18 BL cases had a BI of 1+ or more. All BT and TT cases had a BI of 0.

The prevalence of HIV-1 infection in MB and PB cases of leprosy and population controls by age, sex, and residence is presented in Table 2. HIV-1 prevalence was higher in MB than in PB cases. Overall, the HIV-1 prevalence in leprosy cases was 7 of 72 (10%) in rural, and 2 of 21 (10%) in roadside and urban areas; in controls these prevalences were 3.4% and 9.9% respectively. Of the 7 relapsed cases, 5 had MB leprosy, 1 of whom had HIV-1 infection; the 2 relapsed cases with PB leprosy were HIV-1 negative.

The overall odds ratio for the association between HIV-1 and leprosy that can be calculated from Table 2 was 2.2 (95% CI 1.0–4.7; P=0.07). The odds ratio for the association between HIV-1 and MB leprosy was 4.6 (95% CI = 1.3–13.2; P=0.02); for PB leprosy the odds ratio was 1.4 (95% CI = 0.4–4.7; P=0.72). When relapsed cases are excluded from the analysis the odds ratio for the association between HIV-1 and MB leprosy was 4.1 (95% CI = 1.0–13.3; P=0.06).

The population etiological fraction for the development of MB leprosy can be estimated to be 13% (95% CI = 4–23%). If the association between HIV-1 infection and MB leprosy were causal, 13% of MB leprosy cases occurring at present would be attributable to HIV-1 infection.

Figure 1. Map of Mwanza Region, Tanzania, indicating the residences of identified leprosy cases

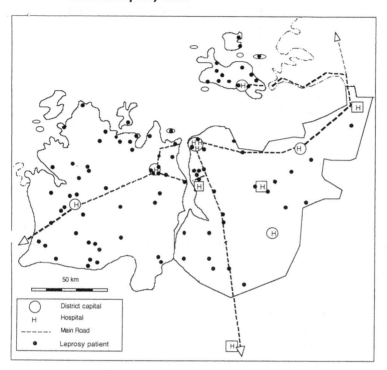

Table 1. Age, sex and residence of leprosy cases and population controls

		Leprosy cases		Population controls	
		Number	(%)	Number	(%)
Age	15-24	12	(13)	1495	(36)
(years)	25-34	27	(29)	1385	(33)
	35-44	35	(38)	770	(19)
	45-54	19	(20)	511	(12)
Sex	Male	61	(66)	2000	(48)
	Female	32	(34)	2161	(52)
Residence	Rural	72	(77)	2019	(49)
	Roadside	18	(19)	958	(23)
	Urban	3	(3)	1184	(28)
Total		93	(100)	4161	(100)

Table 2. HIV-1 prevalence in leprosy cases and population controls by age, sex, and residence

Age group	Multibacillary leprosy		Paucibacillary leprosy		Population controls	
	HIV+/ No. seen	(%)	HIV+/ No. seen	(%)	HIV+/ No. seen	(%)
Rural						
Males						
15-24	0/ 3	(0)	0/ 5	(0)	5/ 314	(1.6)
25-34	4/ 7	(57)	0/ 8	(0)	12/ 309	(3.9)
35-44	0/ 6	(0)	0/ 7	(0)	6/ 191	(3.1)
45-54	0/ 3	(0)	0/ 10	(0)	6/ 160	(3.8)
Subtotal	4/ 19	(21)	0/ 30	(0)	29/ 974	(3.0)
Females						
15-24	0/ 1	(0)	0/ 1	(0)	17/ 397	(4.3)
25-34	1/ 1	(100)	2/ 7	(29)	10/ 330	(3.0)
35-44	0/ 0	(−)	0/ 9	(0)	9/ 210	(4.3)
45-54	0/ 0	(−)	0/ 4	(0)	3/ 108	(2.8)
Subtotal	1/ 2	(50)	2/ 21	(10)	39/ 1045	(3.7)
Total Rural	5/ 21	(24)	2/51	(4)	68/2019	(3.4
Roadside and Urban						
Males						
15-24	0/ 1	(0)	1/ 1	(100)	16/ 356	(4.5)
25-34	0/ 1	(0)	0/ 1	(0)	33/ 340	(9.7)
35-44	0/ 1	(0)	1/ 6	(17)	24/ 200	(12.0)
45-54	0/ 1	(0)	0/ 0	(−)	6/ 130	(4.6)
Subtotal	0/ 4	(0)	2/ 8	(25)	79/ 1026	(7.7)
Females						
15-24	0/ 0	(−)	0/ 0	(−)	56/ 428	(13.1)
25-34	0/ 2	(0)	0/ 0	(−)	61/ 406	(15.0)
35-44	0/ 0	(−)	0/ 6	(0)	13/ 169	(7.7)
45-54	0/ 1	(0)	0/ 0	(−)	3/ 113	(2.7)
Subtotal	0/ 3	(0)	0/ 6	(0)	133/ 1116	(11.9)
Total Roadside and Urban	0/ 7	(0)	2/14	(14)	212/ 2142	(9.9)
Overall total	5/ 28	(18)	4/ 65	(6)	280/ 4161	(6.7)

Discussion

This population-based study has demonstrated an association between HIV-1 infection and the development of MB leprosy in self-reported cases. However, because the number of cases was small, this finding would need to be confirmed in other, if possible, larger studies. An association between HIV-1 infection and MB leprosy theoretically is to be expected, because a reduced cellular immunity, which occurs with the progress of HIV-1 infection, is associated with MB leprosy [7]. It is also expected because of the association between HIV-1 infection and other diseases due to mycobacteria, in particular *M. tuberculosis* [1,4,5,10,12,16].

Comparing self-reported cases with population controls has a danger of introducing a bias, for instance, if health service utilization rather than the disease under study itself were associated with HIV-1 infection. As was done by Pönnighaus, et al. [13], we assessed the validity of the case-control comparison by applying the same methods to a comparison of tuberculosis cases and population controls. The odds ratio for the association between HIV-1 and tuberculosis was 8.3 (95% CI = 6.4–11.0)[18], which is consistent with findings of Pönnighaus, et al. [13] and others [4,5,10]. This provides some support for the validity of the case-control comparison.

For the detection of leprosy cases use was made of passive case finding. Self-reported cases might be expected to show a bias toward more serious cases and toward a residence close to a hospital or a main road. The latter bias is not obvious (The Figure). On the contrary, most leprosy cases were resident in fairly remote rural villages. The clinical presentation and disability grade of HIV-1-infected patients was similar to that of patients without HIV-1 infection. However, because of the possibility of the former bias, our results can be interpreted in two ways: a) an increased incidence of MB leprosy may be attributable to HIV-1 infection or b) HIV-1 infection may contribute to a more serious clinical presentation of leprosy. The odds ratio for the association between MB leprosy and HIV-1 infection has not been influenced much by the inclusion of the relapsed cases.

Another limitation of this study may lie in the classification of leprosy disease. As has been shown elsewhere [3], the concordance between clinical and bacteriological classification was not complete. In particular, 2 of 28 (7%) cases clinically diagnosed as MB (both BL) did not have a positive slit-skin smear result. One of these two was HIV-1 infected. If these two cases were re-classified as PB leprosy, the odds ratio for the association between MB leprosy and HIV-1 infection would be 3.6 (95% CI = 0.9–11.6; P=0.08). The classification of these two cases therefore had some influence on the results obtained. This provides an additional reason for carrying out further studies to confirm the association between HIV-1 and MB leprosy.

The association between HIV-1 infection and leprosy is only apparent in the rural area and not in the urban area or roadside settlements. This may be due to the small number of leprosy patients in the urban area and roadside settlements. The data from these strata have been included for completeness, although they do not contribute much to the final result.

The interaction of HIV-1 and leprosy is difficult to demonstrate because of a number of factors: a) leprosy occurs mainly in the rural areas, while HIV-1 is most prevalent in urban areas; b) the number of new cases of leprosy detected is small in most areas; c) the development of leprosy disease is a slow process, probably taking many years; and d) the loss of immunity in HIV-1 disease is also a slow process, usually taking a number of years to develop. Therefore, future case-control studies aiming at confirming or refuting the association between HIV-1 infection and an increased incidence of leprosy would need to: a) select 'incident' cases of leprosy; b) control for confounders such as age, sex, and residence; c) be carried out in areas where leprosy is fairly common and HIV-1 infection has been well established in the rural areas for a number of years.

All of these criteria were met in the study by Pönnighaus, et al. in Malawi [13] with the exception that HIV-1 had probably been introduced recently in the study area. The studies by Leonard, et al. [8] and Tekle-Haimanot, et al. [17] appear to have had insufficient control for potential confounders, in particular age [8] and residence [17]. The study of Leonard, et al. included some areas where HIV-1 infection had been introduced recently while this is unclear from the study of Tekle-Haimanot, et al. These factors might explain the negative findings of these studies.

The implications of our findings for leprosy control are worrying. In our study 4% to 23% of MB leprosy cases appear to be attributable to HIV-1 infection. If the HIV-1 prevalence increases in the rural areas of the region, the population etiological fraction is likely to increase as well. Over the past 10 years the case detection rate of MB leprosy has been stable, but the numbers are rather small. Hopefully an increase in the incidence of leprosy can be prevented by high cure rates through effective chemotherapy and case holding, by early case detection to limit the infectious period, and by BCG vaccination [9].

Repeating this study elsewhere and in 5 years time in the same location is recommended to assess the impact of HIV-1 infection on the epidemiology and control of leprosy.

Acknowledgment

We thank the Principal Secretary, Kenya Ministry of Health, and the Director-General of the National Institute for Medical Research for permission to carry out and publish the results of this study. We are grateful to the district medical officers, district tuberculosis and leprosy coordinators, and the laboratory staff of the hospitals in the Mwanza Region for their support. Data collection on leprosy cases was financed by the International Union Against Tuberculosis and Lung Diseases and the World Health Organization. The population survey study was financed by the Netherlands Minister for Development Cooperation and the AIDS Task Force of the European Community. We thank Prof. A. S. Muller, Dr. J. Velema, and Dr. W. Deville for critically reviewing the manuscript.

References

1. American Thoracic Society. Mycobacterioses and the acquired immune deficiency syndrome. Am. Rev. Respir. Dis. 136 (1987) 492-496.
2. Barongo, L.R., Borgdorff, M.W., Mosha, F.F., Nicoll, A., Grosskurth, H., Senkoro, K.P., Newell, J.N., Changalucha, J., Klokke, A.H., Killewo, J.Z., et al. The epidemiology of HIV-1 infection in urban areas, roadside settlements and rural villages in Mwanza Region, Tanzania. AIDS 6 (1992) 1521-1528.
3. Becx-Bleumink, M. Allocation of patients to paucibacillary or multibacillary drug regimens for the treatment of leprosy: a comparison of methods based mainly on skin smears as opposed to clinical methods; Alternative clinical methods for classification of patients. Int. J. Lepr. 59 (1991) 292-303.
4. Braun, M.M., Badi, N., Ryder, R.W., Baende, E., Mukade, Y., Nsuami, M., Matela, B., Williame, J.C., Kaboto, M. and Heyward, W. A retrospective cohort study of the risk of tuberculosis among women of childbearing age with HIV infection in Zaire. Am. Rev. Respir. Dis. 143 (1991) 501-504.
5. De Cock, K.M., Gnaore, E., Adjorlolo, G., Braun, M.M., Lafontaine, M.F., Yesso, G., Bretton, G., Coulibaly, I.M., Gershy-Damet, G.M., Bretton, R., et al. Risk of tuberculosis in patients with HIV-I and HIV-II infections in Abidjan, Ivory Coast. BMJ 302 (1991) 496-499.
6. Dharmendra. Classifications of leprosy. In: Leprosy. Hastings, R.C., ed. Edinburgh: Churchill Livingstone, 1985, pp. 88-99.
7. Harboe, M. The immunology of leprosy. In: Leprosy. Hastings, R.C., ed. Edinburgh: Churchill Livingstone, 1985, pp. 53-87.
8. Leonard, G., Sangare, A., Verdier, M., Sassou-Guesseau, E., Petit, G., Milan, J., M'Boup, S., Rey, J.L., Dumas, J.L., Hugon, J., et al. Prevalence of HIV infection among patients with leprosy in African countries and Yemen. J. Acquir. Immune Defic. Syndr. 3 (1990) 1109-1113.
9. Lienhardt, C. and Fine, P.E.M. Controlling leprosy. BMJ 305 (1992) 206-207.
10. Long, R., Scalcini, M., Manfreda, J., Carre, G., Philippe E., Hershfield, E., Sekla, L. and Stachiw, W. Impact of human immunodeficiency virus type 1 on tuberculosis in rural Haiti. Am. Rev. Respir. Dis. 143 (1991) 69-73.
11. Meeran, K. Prevalence of HIV infection among patients with leprosy and tuberculosis in rural Zambia. BMJ 298 (1989) 364-365.
12. Pitchenik, A.E. The treatment and prevention of mycobacterial disease in patients with HIV infection. AIDS 2 Suppl. 1 (1988) S177-S182.
13. Pönnighaus J.M., Mwanjasi, L.J., Fine, P.E.M., Shaw, M.-A., Turner, A.C., Oxborrow, S.M., Lucas, S.B., Jenkins, P.A., Sterne, J.A.C. and Bliss, L. Is HIV infection a risk factor for leprosy? Int. J. Lepr. 59 (1992) 221-228.
14. Rees, R.J.W. The microbiology of leprosy. In: Leprosy. Hastings, R.C., ed. Edinburgh: Churchill Livingstone, 1985, pp. 31-52.
15. Schlesselman, J.J. Case-Control Studies - Design, Conduct, Analysis. Oxford: Oxford University Press, 1982, pp. 220-226.
16. Selwyn, P.A., Hartel, D., Lewis, V.A., Schoenbaum, E.E., Vermund, S.H., Klein, R.S., Walker, A.T., and Friedland, G.H. A prospective study of the risk of tuberculosis among intravenous drug users with human immunodeficiency virus infection. N. Engl. J. Med. 320 (1989) 545-550.
17. Tekle-Haimanot, R., Frommel, D., Tadesse, T., Verdier, M., Abebe, M., and Denis, F. A survey of HTLV-1 and HIVs in Ethiopian leprosy patients. AIDS 5 (1991) 108-110.

18. Van den Broek, J., Borgdorff, M.W., Pakker, N.G., et al. HIV-1 infection as a risk factor for the development of tuberculosis disease: a population-based case-control study in Tanzania. Int. J. Epidemiol. 1993; 22:1159-1165.
19. WHO Expert Committee on Leprosy. Sixth Report. Geneva: World Health Organization, 1988. Tech. Rep. Ser. 768.
20. WHO Study Group. Chemotherapy of leprosy for control programmes. Geneva: World Health Organization, 1982. Tech. Rep. Ser. 675.
21. WHO Study Group. Epidemiology of leprosy in relation to control. Geneva: World Health Organization, 1985. Tech. Rep. Ser. 716.
22. World Health Organization. Acquired immune deficiency syndrome (AIDS) - Proposed WHO criteria for interpreting results from Western blot assays for HIV-1, HIV-2, and HTLV-I/HTLV-II. Wkly. Epidemiol. Rec. 65 (1990) 281-283.

7

The establishment of a cohort study of urban factory workers and results at intake

Preparing a cohort study of urban factory workers

After completion of the population survey (Chapter 3), we started a cohort study of factory workers and their spouses in Mwanza Municipality, in order to determine the incidence of HIV-1 and other sexually transmitted diseases and identify risk factors for HIV-1 seroconversion and for contracting other sexually transmitted diseases. Another objective was to document changes in risk behaviour, in particular condom use and partner change, and determine whether these were associated with a reduced incidence of HIV-1 and other sexually transmitted diseases. Finally, the cohort study aimed at providing information on the natural history of HIV-1 infection.

When the plans for the cohort study were first formulated, it was envisaged that the study would be carried out as an interdisciplinary effort with particularly close collaboration between epidemiologists and social scientists in the study of sexual risk behaviour. The study site was originally planned to be a textile factory. When the research proposals were developed in more detail in November 1989, an occupational cohort was considered to be potentially problematic, in view of experiences with such studies in Dar es Salaam (maintaining confidentiality of HIV results appeared to be a particular problem). Therefore, it was decided to carry out a community-based study instead, despite the much greater demand this would involve in following up individuals over time.

When the population survey was carried out, tracing people at their homes in the urban areas proved indeed to be difficult and time consuming. In order to ensure high rates of follow-up, it was therefore decided to explore the possibilities for an occupational cohort study once more. An inventory was made of large employers, and a textile factory was provisionally selected as it was the workplace with the largest number of employees on a single site (between 1,500 and 2,000). A major drawback was that the majority of those employees were male. A large number of female employees were present in the referral hospital, but this site was not selected because confidentiality would be much more difficult to maintain (HIV testing took place in the same hospital), and because the incentive to participate (free medical care) would be much less valuable to the paramedical staff concerned. Civil servants might have been selected as a large proportion of them are women, but in the early stages this was thought to be risky politically.

The management of the textile factory was approached: it was positive towards the proposal of a study. As a next step brief meetings were organized by the management between the researchers and groups of approximately 30 workers at a time. In one day approximately 600 workers were seen at such meetings. At these meetings the aims and activities of the proposed study were explained, after which all those present were requested to complete an anonymous, self-administered questionnaire, which sought information on their willingness to participate in the proposed study, in particular when it concerned taking blood, urine, and stool samples. Over 90% of workers present at those meetings gave a positive response. However, another problem arose: in this period the factory was closed for a couple of weeks due to financial problems, and the management was replaced. Thereafter, the factory appeared to be operating fairly satisfactory, so we decided to continue there, as no better alternatives appeared to be available.

At the factory a clinic provided free health care to factory staff and their spouses and children. The number of staff and facilities available were limited because of financial constraints. The building was too small to cope with additional staff. Therefore, the researchers preferred to set up an additional clinic on the factory grounds. (This was supported by the factory management which made rooms available that the project converted into a study clinic). The clinic was open for the staff themselves (and after 15 weeks also for their spouses). The children of staff continued to attend the existing factory clinic and were not included in the studies. The study clinic was advertised through the meetings mentioned above, and thereafter through the management and noticeboards.

In order to learn from the experience of others in setting up a cohort study, the two epidemiologists in charge of the cohort study visited the Medical Research Council's Research Programme in Uganda, which proved to be very valuable.

Development of the main questionnaire and training of interviewers were undertaken together. First, a draft questionnaire was prepared in English. This was discussed and translated, involving social scientists in the project and the interviewers. The interviewers were paramedical staff, largely selected from the ones involved in the population survey (Chapter 3), and seconded by the Regional Medical Officer and Medical Officer of Health. The Swahili version was pre-tested and adjusted twice, which led to minor clarifications in many questions, a reordering of questions (putting the more sensitive ones on sexual techniques at the end), and omitting questions on oral-genital sexual contact which were felt to be embarrassing or insulting by some respondents. The interviewers were initially a bit shy when interviewing people about sexual behaviour, and the pre-testing period was useful to overcome this.

A similar training and pre-testing period was undertaken with the laboratory staff in order to standardize and clarify procedures, both in performing laboratory tests and in the handling and storage of samples and results. The STD laboratory (microbiology and serology) was based in the National Institute for Medical Research, Mwanza Centre, and the HIV laboratory in Bugando Medical Centre.

Assistant Medical Officers were recruited to carry out the physical examinations and prescribe treatment where necessary. Training in carrying out the physical examination was given on the spot (in the study clinic) by the two epidemiologists. A trained nurse-counsellor was recruited, who first prepared and discussed guidelines for counselling, and then started her work at the factory. All individuals were asked at the end of the interview whether they agreed to bloodletting for STD/HIV testing, and if they did, whether they wished to be informed of their HIV result. Those that expressed an interest in knowing their HIV result were asked to see a counsellor, who discussed the pros and cons of knowing one's HIV status with the clients. From those still interested in knowing their HIV test result, a separate sample of blood was taken and tested under a different code number: only the counsellor knew which person belonged to this second code number. This ensured confidentiality, and also provided a blinded internal quality control of HIV testing.

The flow and storage of information and samples form a vital aspect of a cohort study. Procedures regarding the flow and storage of information were thought out and prepared as much as possible in advance, making use of experience in the Amsterdam cohort studies. They continued to need a lot of attention in the initial stages. The registration office at the study clinic, manned by a competent and conscientious statistical assistant (who had completed four years of secondary school and thereafter received the on the job training), played a particularly important role in data handling at the clinic. Managing the follow up of study participants who do not return spontaneously, ensuring that those attending the clinic attend at all relevant stations (interview, examination, counselling, laboratory) and avoiding loss of information such as completed questionnaires, all require a conscientious 'data manager' at the clinic, who is good in handling people at the same time.

A special point of attention was the use of code numbers for individuals. These were needed to uniquely and consistently identify individuals over time in order allow linkage of all information on each subject. Code numbers were also needed to ensure confidentiality of HIV test results. Although the factory used code numbers to identify their employees, these were sometimes changed and therefore unsuitable for research purposes; anonymity could also not be ensured with these. The project adopted a simple coding system using sequential 4-digit numbers with a 5th check digit to easily trace the majority of copying errors. At the registration office lists were kept of study numbers, factory numbers, and names of study participants to make it easy to trace study numbers when study participants presented with the card the project had issued to them on registration with their name and factory number.

Another issue was the organization of follow-up. All study participants were invited for follow-up visits four months (17 weeks) after their previous visit. A follow-up worker reminded them of their appointment the week before. If they did not attend, they were re-invited at 22 weeks, 27 weeks, and 42 weeks. At 50 weeks they would receive a letter informing them that unless they attended within the next two weeks, they would no longer be considered a study participant. In order to trace conveniently the week of follow-up in which various participants were, registration cards were kept according to week number of next appointment.

All data entry took place at the National Institute for Medical Research, Mwanza Centre, and only minimal data (necessary for follow-up and medical treatment) were kept at the clinic. This proved convenient in data processing (entry and cleaning) and made it also easy to maintain confidentiality and 'blinding' of research staff at the clinic. One disadvantage might be that information on individuals is not linked continuously, making it harder to spot inconsistencies early on.

It took a long time before all equipment ordered for the study arrived, largely because there was a delay in decision making on funding of the second phase of the project. This resulted in some equipment such as weight and height measuring scales arriving as late as half a year after the start of the study.

After all these preparations a one week pilot study was conducted at the factory to identify final problems. This led to a period of adjustment of questionnaires and procedures, after which the study fully started in October 1991.

The following section of this chapter (also published separately) reports on findings at intake with respect to risk factors for HIV-1 infection.

Intake of a cohort study of urban factory workers in Northwest Tanzania: Risk factors for HIV–1 infection

L.R. Barongo[1], M.W. Borgdorff[1,3], J.N. Newell[1], K.P. Senkoro[1], A.H. Klokke[2], J. Changalucha[1], W. Deville[3], J.P. Velema[4], R.A. Coutinho[5], R.M. Gabone[1]

Tropical and Geographical Medicine 1994; 46: 157-162

Summary

A cohort study has been started of urban factory workers and their spouses in Tanzania, in order to 1) identify risk factors for HIV–1 seroconversion, and 2) document changes over time in risk behaviour, in particular condom use and partner change, and determine whether these are associated with a reduced incidence of HIV–1 and other sexually transmitted diseases. We report findings at intake from October 1991 to March 1992. Study participants were interviewed, examined, and screened for HIV–1 and syphilis. HIV–1 prevalence was 91/926 (10%) in males and 36/217 (17%) in females. Statistically significant risk factors for HIV–1 infection in males were age group, region of birth, not being married for more than 5 years, being uncircumcised, having had a genital ulcer in the past four months, and having received injections from medical staff in the past four months. HIV–1 incidence in this group is expected to be between 1% and 2% per year. It is concluded that a longitudinal study is needed to assess the importance of partner change. This cohort appears to be suitable for such a study as HIV–1 incidence is expected to be fairly high, HIV–1 prevalence and risk factors are comparable to those of the general population and cooperation of the factory workers is good.

1 National Institute for Medical Research, Mwanza, Tanzania
2 Bugando Medical Centre, Mwanza, Tanzania
3 Royal Tropical Institute, Amsterdam, The Netherlands
4 Nijmegen Institute for International Health, Nijmegen, The Netherlands
5 Municipal Health Service, Amsterdam, The Netherlands

Introduction

HIV–1 infection has a higher prevalence in urban than in rural areas in many countries [1,2], as have other sexually transmitted diseases. [3,4] A higher rate of partner change in urban than in rural areas may be an important determinant of this increased prevalence. [5,6] In a population-based survey in Mwanza Region, Northwest Tanzania, HIV–1 prevalence in the age group 15–54 years was found to be 11.8% in the urban area, 7.3% in villages along the main roads and 2.5% in rural villages. [7] Risk factors most strongly associated with risk of HIV–1 infection were being separated or widowed in males, and for females having had more than one formal or informal marriage in the past five years.

After completion of the population survey, we started a cohort study of factory workers and their spouses in Mwanza Municipality in order to identify risk factors for HIV–1 seroconversion and for contracting other sexually transmitted diseases with special regard to partner change. Another objective was to document changes in risk behaviour, in particular condom use and partner change, and determine whether these are associated with a reduced incidence of HIV–1 and other sexually transmitted diseases.

In this paper the findings at intake are reported on risk factors for HIV–1 infection. This intake took place from October 1991 to March 1992. The main aim of this analysis was to determine the suitability of this group for further follow-up in a cohort study. The findings on determinants of condom use and partner change will be reported separately.

Subjects and methods

Study population
The study population comprised workers and their spouses at a large urban factory with a work force of 1,728 workers, 13% of whom were female. Workers were enroled from the start, spouses from 15 weeks after the start of the study. A study clinic was created at the factory in addition to an existing clinic, as the latter was too small to cope with additional activities. Prior to starting the study, the willingness of the study population to participate was determined through an anonymous, self-administered questionnaire which produced a positive response of more than 90%. The study population has been advised that the aim of the study is to determine the health status of the workers, with special interest in sexually transmitted diseases and HIV–1 infection.

Data collection techniques
All respondents were interviewed for 30 to 45 minutes in Swahili by trained inter-viewers, using a structured and pre-coded questionnaire. All women were interviewed by a female interviewer, most of the men by a male interviewer. A physical exam-ination was then carried out by an assistant medical officer. Those reporting the presence of a genital discharge, genital ulcer, or lower abdominal pain, underwent a genital examination.

From all study participants 10 ml of venous blood was taken using a vacuum system, and the blood sample was separated in the study clinic.

Serum was tested for HIV–1 antibodies with the Vironostika anti-HTLV–III ELISA (Organon, Boxtel, The Netherlands). All non-negative samples underwent confirmatory testing using Western Blot (Organon, Epitope, Beaverton, Oregon, USA). The Western Blot was considered positive if at least two of the gp41, gp120, and gp160 bands were present. [8] To diagnose syphilis infection a Treponema Pallidum Haemagglutination test (TPHA, Organon, Boxtel, The Netherlands) was performed, followed by a Rapid Plasma Reagin (RPR) test (Organon, Boxtel, The Netherlands) on sera with a positive TPHA result. A positive TPHA with a positive RPR was interpreted as indicating active or recently treated syphilis infection, while a positive TPHA and negative RPR was interpreted as a cured syphilis infection. [9]

Counselling and treatment
Pre- and post-HIV-test counselling was offered to all. Pre-test counselling was given to 332 (30%) of study participants. Of these, 148 (45%) returned for post-test counselling. After pre-test counselling a separate blood sample was sent to the laboratory, the result of which was made known to the counsellor only. Other staff at the factory clinic were blind to the HIV–1 status of individuals.

Free medical treatment was provided to all study participants. Where necessary, patients were referred to the hospital for further investigation or treatment.

Data analysis
Age adjusted odds ratios (OR) and their 95% confidence intervals (CI) were calculated using the Mantel-Haenszel method. Logistic regression was used to simultaneously adjust for various variables of interest. Variables were included in the regression model if they showed a significant association with HIV–1 infection on univariate analysis or for a priori reasons (e.g. marital status).

Results

In the first 19 weeks of the study 1,096 workers (926 male, 170 female) and 47 spouses (all female) were enroled. These workers comprised 62% of the male and 76% of the female work force.

Prevalence of HIV–1 infection, syphilis, genital ulcers, and genital discharge
HIV–1 prevalence was 91/926 (10%) in males, and 36/217 (17%) in females (χ^2 =7.47, $P<0.01$). The difference in HIV–1 prevalence between female employees (31/170 = 18%) and spouses (5/47 = 11%) was not significant (χ^2 =1.0, $P>0.05$). HIV–1 was most prevalent in those aged 25–44, both in men and women (table 1). The HIV prevalence by age in men aged less than 30 years is presented in the figure. It shows a mean increase in the prevalence of HIV–1 of 1.4% per year of age.

Serologically defined untreated or recently treated syphilis was found in 8%, while another 6% had evidence of a cured syphilis infection (table 2). Eighteen per cent of male and 7% of female respondents reported ever having had a genital ulcer (OR 2.7,

Figure   HIV-1 prevalence by age in 269 male urban factory workers aged 15-29 years

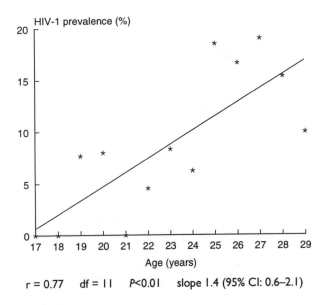

r = 0.77   df = 11   P<0.01   slope 1.4 (95% CI: 0.6–2.1)

95% CI: 1.6–4.7), while 45% of males and 12% of females had ever had a genital discharge (OR 5.7, 95% CI: 3.7–8.7). The reported incidence of genital ulcer and genital discharge over the past four months were 3% and 6% re- spectively with little difference between the sexes.

The following proportions of reported sexually transmitted disease syndromes were confirmed at examination: genital ulcer in men 10/11 (91%), genital discharge in men 15/24 (63%), genital ulcer in women 0/2 (0%) and genital discharge in women 6/6 (100%).

Risk factors for HIV–1 infection
HIV–1 prevalence by risk factor in males is given in table 3. The following risk factors may be distinguished (the odds ratios given below are adjusted for age).
HIV–1 prevalence was higher in those born in Kagera, a neighbouring Region (OR 3.1). It was not associated with the Region in which respondents had lived prior to coming to Mwanza.

HIV–1 infection tended to be more common in men being separated, widowed, or living apart from their spouse than in married or single (never married) men (OR 2.1, P=0.12). It was significantly more common in those who had had at least one separa- tion per 10 years of being married (OR 2.3). It was also more common in those who were not married at interview (OR 2.2) or who had been married for less than five years (OR 3.1), than in those married for five years or more. Those who lived in a large size household and those with five or more children had a decreased HIV prevalence (OR 0.4 in each group).

Table 1 HIV–1 prevalence by age and sex in 1,096 urban factory workers and 47 female spouses in Tanzania

Age (years)	Male HIV+/No. seen	%	Female HIV+/No. seen	%	Total HIV+/No. seen	%
15–24	8/ 146	5	7/ 67	10	15/ 214	7
25–34	42/ 297	14	20/ 99	20	62/ 396	16
35–44	35/ 350	10	8/ 41	20	43/ 390	11
45–54	6/ 120	5	1/ 10	10	7/ 130	5
≥55	0/ 13	0	–	–	0/ 13	0
Total	91/ 926	10	36/ 217	17	127/ 1143	11

Table 2 Prevalence of syphilis and reported prevalence and incidence of genital ulcers and genital discharge in 1,096 urban factory workers and 46 female spouses in Tanzania

	Male No. cases/ total	%	Female No. cases/ total	%	Total No. cases/ total	%
Syphilis *						
Untreated or recently treated	80/ 921	9	7/ 215	3	87/ 1136	8
Cured	55/ 921	6	9/ 215	4	64/ 1136	6
Genital ulcer						
Now	15/ 925	2	2/ 217	1	17/ 1142	1
Within past 4 months	27/ 923	3	8/ 217	4	35/ 1140	3
Ever	165/ 923	18	16/ 216	7	181/ 1139	16
Genital discharge						
Now	30/ 926	3	8/ 217	4	38/ 1143	3
Within past 4 months	51/ 924	6	16/ 217	7	67/ 1141	6
Ever	415/ 926	45	27/ 217	12	442/ 1143	39

* Untreated or recently treated: TPHA+ and RPR+; cured syphilis: TPHA+ and RPR–

Table 3 HIV-1 prevalence by risk factor in 926 male urban factory workers

Risk factor	No. infected/ No. seen	%	Crude OR (95% CI)		OR adjusted for age (95% CI)	
Age group						
15–24	8/ 146	5	1	p<0.005	–	
25–34	42/ 297	14	2.8	(1.2–6.8)	–	
35–44	35/ 350	10	1.9	(0.8–4.6)	–	
45–64	6/ 133	5	0.8	(0.3–2.7)	–	
Year started work at factory						
<1980	32/ 443	7	1	p=0.01	1	p=0.01
≥1980	59/ 480	12	1.8	(1.1–2.9)	2.0	(1.1–3.7)
Birthplace						
Mwanza	60/ 557	11	1	p<0.01	1	p<0.01
Shinyanga/Mara	11/ 164	7	0.6	(0.3–1.2)	0.6	(0.3–1.2)
Kagera	9/ 39	23	2.5	(1.0–5.8)	3.1	(1.3–7.8)
Other	11/ 166	7	0.6	(0.3–1.2)	0.6	(0.3–1.2)
Marital status						
Married	69/ 717	10	1	p<0.1	1	p=0.12
Single	12/ 155	8	0.8	(0.4–1.6)	1.0	(0.4–2.4)
Separated*	10/ 54	19	2.1	(1.0–4.6)	2.1	(1.0–4.7)
Separation rate †						
0–	53/ 635	8	1	p<0.001	1	p<0.01
1+	25/ 127	20	2.7	(1.6–4.7)	2.3	(1.3–4.1)
Never married	12/ 155	8	0.9	(0.5–1.8)	1.1	(0.4–2.7)
Number of years married with present spouse						
≥5	39/ 567	7	1	p<0.001	1	p<0.001
<5	30/ 149	20	3.4	(2.0–5.9)	3.1	(1.8–6.1)
Unmarried now	22/ 209	11	1.6	(0.9–2.9)	2.2	(1.2–5.3)
Household size						
≥5	40/ 611	7	1	p<0.001	1	p<0.001
<5	51/ 315	16	2.8	(1.7–4.4)	2.8	(1.8–5.0)
Number of children						
0–4	74/ 613	12	1	p<0.01	1	p<0.01
≥5	17/ 310	5	0.4	(0.2–0.8)	0.4	(0.2–0.8)

Table 3, continued

Risk factor	No. infected/ No. seen	%	Crude OR (95% CI)		OR adjusted for age (95% CI)	
Injections from medical staff						
0	40/ 585	7	1	p<0.001	1	p<0.001
1–4	21/ 156	13	2.1	(1.2–3.8)	2.1	(1.2–3.9)
≥5	30/ 185	16	2.6	(1.5–4.5)	2.7	(1.6–4.6)
Circumcision						
Yes	24/ 432	6	1	p<0.001	1	p<0.001
No	67/ 494	14	2.7	(1.6–4.5)	2.6	(1.6–4.4)
Genital discharge last						
Never	38/ 511	7	1	p<0.05	1	p<0.1
≥4 months	45/ 362	12	1.8	(1.1–2.9)	1.6	(1.0–2.7)
<4 months	3/ 21	14	2.1	(0.5–7.9)	2.3	(0.5–9.3)
Now	5/ 30	17	2.5	(0.8–7.4)	2.3	(0.8–7.4)
Genital discharge treated						
Yes	49/ 401	12	1	p<0.05	1	p<0.05
No	4/ 11	36	4.1	(1.0–16.4)	3.7	(1.0–18.2)
Genital ulcer last						
Never	59/ 758	8	1	p<0.001	1	p<0.001
≥4 months	28/ 136	21	2.0	(1.1–3.6)	1.9	(1.0–3.3)
<4 months	6/ 12	50	11.9	(3.3–43.1)	12.0	(3.3–46.5)
Now	6/ 15	40	7.9	(2.4–25.3)	8.6	(2.4–28.1)
Genital ulcer treated						
Yes	28/ 148	19	1	p>0.4	1	p>0.4
No	4/ 15	27	1.6	(0.4–5.9)	1.6	(0.4–6.3)
Syphilis						
Never	71/ 786	9	1	p<0.1	1	p<0.1
Treated	7/ 55	13	1.5	(0.6–3.5)	1.4	(0.6–3.5)
Active	13/ 80	16	2.0	(1.0–3.9)	2.0	(1.0–3.9)

* Separated includes married but living apart, and widowed
† 10 x (Number of separations)/(Number of years being married)

Table 4   Odds ratios of risk factors for HIV infection in 926 male factory workers adjusted for factors of interest* using logistic regression

Risk factor	Adjusted OR	(95% CI)
Age group		
15–24	1	
25–34	4.2	(1.6–11.3)
35–44	3.9	(1.3–11.5)
45–54	1.8	(0.5–6.7)
Birthplace		
Mwanza	1	
Shinyanga/Mara	0.9	(0.4–2.0)
Kagera	4.1	(1.7–10.1)
Other	0.8	(0.4–1.7)
Marital status		
Married ≥5 years †	1	
Married <5 years †	3.3	(1.8–6.1)
Separated/widowed	2.7	(1.2–6.3)
Single	1.8	(0.7–4.7)
Circumcision		
Yes	1	
No	2.5	(1.4–4.4)
Injections from medical staff		
0	1	
1–4	2.5	(1.4–4.6)
≥5	2.2	(1.3–3.9)
Genital ulcer last		
Never	1	
>4 months	1.6	(0.9–2.9)
<4 months	9.1	(2.5–33.3)
Now	5.4	(1.7–17.6)

* Adjusted for age group, birth place, marital status (including years being married with present spouse), circumcision, injections from medical staff, and genital ulcers
† Duration of being married with current spouse

No association was found between HIV–1 infection and indicators of recent partner change, such as having had multiple sexual partners in the past month. Also no association was found between HIV–1 infection and age at first sexual intercourse nor with practising other sexual techniques than heterosexual vaginal intercourse. Around 5% of respondents reported that they practised other sexual techniques.

HIV–1 infection was more common in uncircumcised than in circumcised men (OR 2.6). All except 5 of the 77 muslim men were circumcised. In the non-muslims the OR for lack of circumcision was 2.5 (95% CI: 1.5–4.4).

HIV–1 infection was more prevalent in those with a reported genital ulcer or genital discharge (past or present); among men having had a genital discharge it was more prevalent in those who did not seek treatment for it. HIV–1 tended to be more common (p<0.1) in those with serological evidence of syphilis.

Blood transfusions and scarifications were little reported and showed no association with HIV–1 infection. In those reporting having received one or more injections in the past four months HIV–1 prevalence was increased (1–4 injections, OR 2.1; 5+ injections, OR 2.7).

The factors indicating significantly increased risk after logistic regression were age group, being born in Kagera, not being married for more than five years, being uncircumcised, having had a genital ulcer in the past four months or at intake, and having received injections from medical staff in the past four months (table 4). Univariate analysis showed a similar pattern of risk factors for women, but not all of these were significant, and their numbers were too small for multivariate analysis.

Discussion

This study shows that HIV–1 prevalence in this cohort of factory workers was quite high at 11% and comparable to that of the general population of the town concerned. [7] The mean increase of HIV prevalence with age in those below 30 years of age was 1.4% per year, providing a rough estimate of the incidence that may be expected in the future in this group.

The risk factors which have been identified in this group of factory workers were similar to those found in the general urban population [7] and to those found in other studies. [10–17] They were age, birth place, number of years having been married to the current spouse, having had a genital ulcer, and having received injections from medical staff. However, contrary to earlier findings in this region [7], circumcision was now also found to be strongly associated with a reduced HIV–1 prevalence: adjusting for religion did not affect this conclusion.

Conflicting results on the association of HIV–1 and circumcision have been reported from other countries: in Nairobi, Kenya, and Abidjan, Ivory Coast, a strong association was found between lack of circumcision and HIV–1 infection [14–16], but this was not the case in Rwanda. [17] The role of circumcision in protecting against HIV–1 infection is still unclear, and no final conclusion seems possible at this stage. It is interesting to note that in this study circumcised men were twice as likely to have used condoms than uncircumcised men.

Kagera is a neighbouring region which borders Rwanda and Uganda. It was from Kagera that the first AIDS cases in Tanzania were reported in 1983 and HIV–1 prevalence is known to be high. [5] Being born in Kagera was a risk factor, but having lived in Kagera prior to coming to Mwanza was not. This may imply that people born in Kagera have high risk sexual behaviour, while visitors to Kagera have not, or that the risk for visitors of getting infected in Kagera is at present not much higher than elsewhere in the country, because people take precautions in this recognized high risk area.

In the present study questions about sexual contacts with marital partners, steady partners, and casual partners were asked only for the past month, as bias was expected to be large for a longer recall period. No association was found between indicators of recent partner change and HIV–1 infection. The reported numbers of various types of partners appeared to be fairly reliable. Having had multiple partners in the past month was reported by a large proportion of respondents (28%) and was associated with having had a recent genital discharge (data not shown). The impression of the interviewers was that people were at ease answering questions on partner relations. However, as most HIV–1 infections would have been acquired before the recall period of one month, recent partner change would have to be a good indicator of past partner change to show an association with HIV–1 infection. Follow-up is expected to provide more information on this.

Whereas respondents appeared to be at ease answering questions on partner relations, questions on sexual techniques were sometimes met with embarrassment. Practices such as anal intercourse and sexual intercourse during the menstrual period were possibly underreported.

Some of the risk factors identified may be consequences of HIV–1 infection rather than contributing factors. For instance, HIV–1 infected individuals may be more likely to receive injections for various illness episodes [17], and probably suffer more frequently from genital ulcers than those not infected with HIV–1. [3] However, not adjusting for these two risk factors in logistic regression makes little difference to the results in table 4. The temporal association between these variables and HIV–1 infection will be assessed in the longitudinal study.

We conclude that to assess the importance of the various risk factors, in particular those concerning partner change, a longitudinal study is necessary. This cohort appears to be suitable for such a study as 1) HIV–1 incidence is expected to be fairly high, 2) HIV–1 prevalence and risk factors appear to be comparable to those in the general population, 3) cooperation of the factory workers has been good, and 4) follow-up should be relatively easy in this occupational cohort.

Acknowledgements

We thank the Principal Secretary, Ministry of Health, and the Director General, National Institute for Medical Research, for permission to carry out the study and to publish its results. We thank Prof. A.S. Muller for critically reviewing the manuscript.
The research for this publication was financed by the Netherlands' Minister for Development Cooperation, Section for Research and Technology, P.O. Box 20061, 2500 EB, The Hague, The Netherlands, as part of the Tanzania-Netherlands Research Project on AIDS and HIV Infection in Mwanza Region. Responsibility for the contents and for the opinions expressed rests solely with the authors; publication does not constitute an endorsement by the Netherlands' Minister for Development Cooperation.

References

1. Piot P, Plummer FA, Mhalu FS, Lamboray JL, Chin J, Mann JM. AIDS: an international perspective. Science 1988;239:573-9

2. Rwandan HIV seroprevalence study group. Nationwide community-based serological survey of HIV-1 and other human retrovirus infections in a Central African country. Lancet 1989;i:941-3

3. Laga M, Nzila N, Goeman J. The interrelationship of sexually transmitted diseases and HIV infection: implications for the control of both epidemics in Africa. AIDS 1991;5(suppl 1):S55-S63

4. Piot P, Laga M, Ryder R, et al. The global epidemiology of HIV infection: continuity, heterogeneity, and change. J Acq Imm Def Syndr 1990;3:403-12

5. Killewo J, Nyamuryekung'e K, Sandström A, et al. Prevalence of HIV-1 infection in the Kagera region of Tanzania: a population-based study. AIDS 1990;4:1081-5

6. Serwadda D, Wawer MJ, Musgrave SD, Sewankambo NK, Kaplan JE, Gray RH. HIV risk factors in three geographic strata of rural Rakai District, Uganda. AIDS 1992;6:983-9

7. Barongo LR, Borgdorff MW, Mosha FF, et al. The epidemiology of HIV-1 infection in urban areas, roadside settlements and rural villages in Mwanza Region, Tanzania. AIDS 1992;6:1521-8

8. World Health Organization. Acquired Immune Deficiency Syndrome (AIDS) - Proposed WHO criteria for interpreting results from Western blot assays for HIV-1, HIV-2, and HTLV-I/HTLV-II. Wkly Epid Rec 1990;65:281-3

9. Adler MW. ABC of sexually transmitted diseases. London: British Medical Association, 1984.

10. Ryder RW, Ndilu M, Hassig SE, et al. Heterosexual transmission of HIV-1 among employees and their spouses at two large businesses in Zaire. AIDS 1990;4:725-32

11. Allen S, Lindan C, Serufilira A, et al. Human immunodeficiency virus infection in Rwanda. Demographic and behavioral correlates in a representative sample of childbearing women. JAMA 1991;266:1657-63

12. Bassett MT, Latif AS, Katzenstein DA, Emmanuel JC. Sexual behaviour and risk factors for HIV infection in a group of male factory workers who donated blood in Harare, Zimbabwe. J Acq Imm Def Syndr 1992;5:556-9

13. Nzila N, Laga M, Thiam MA, et al. HIV and other sexually transmitted diseases among female prostitutes in Kinshasa. AIDS 1991;5:715-21

14. Cameron DW, Simonsen JN, D'Costa LJ, et al. Female to male transmission of human immunodeficiency virus type 1: risk factors for seroconversion in men. Lancet 1989;ii:403-7

15. Simonsen JN, Cameron DW, Gakinya MN, et al. Human immunodeficiency virus infection among men with sexually transmitted diseases - Experience from a center in Africa. New Engl J Med 1988;319:274-8

16. Diallo MO, Ackah AN, Lafontaine MF, et al. HIV-1 and HIV-2 infections in men attending sexually transmitted diseases clinics in Abidjan, Côte d'Ivoire. AIDS 1992;6:581-5

17. Van de Perre P, Carael M, Nzaramba D, Zissis G, Kayihigi J, Butzler J. Risk factors for HIV seropositivity in selected urban-based Rwandese adults. AIDS 1987;1:207-11

8

Sexual partner change and condom use among urban factory workers in northwest Tanzania

Martien W Borgdorff[1,2], Longin R Barongo[1], James N Newell[1], Kesheni P Senkoro[1] Walter Deville[2], Johan P Velema[3], RM Gabone

Genitourinary Medicine, 1994, in press

Summary

Objective. To describe sexual partner change and condom use at the intake of a cohort study of urban factory workers in Tanzania.

Methods. From October 1991 to March 1992, 926 male and 170 female factory workers were interviewed using a structured, pre-coded questionnaire. Questionnaire reliability was assessed by pre-testing and comparison with results of unstructured interviews and carrying out repeat questionnaires on a sub-sample.

Results. Almost half of both men and women had had sexual intercourse by their 17th birthday. The period of premarital sex had an interquartile range of 2 to 10 years in men and 0 to 2.5 years in women. Having had sexual intercourse in the past month with more than one partner was reported by 22% of the men and 5% of the women. Factors associated with multiple partners in men were being born in or near Mwanza Region, having low education and low income, and being married. Condoms had been used in the past month by 3% only, mainly with casual partners. Condom use in men was associated with being young, living in town, being born in Kagera Region, high education and high income, being circumcised, and having casual or steady (non-marital) partners.

Conclusion. Information, education and communication (IEC) on sexual relationships and condom use should start at an early age, and include education at primary schools. Much sexual partner change appears to occur through steady (non-marital) partnerships, indicating the need for IEC to be expanded beyond groups such as commercial sex workers and their clients.

1 National Institute for Medical Research, Mwanza, Tanzania
2 Royal Tropical Institute, Amsterdam, The Netherlands
3 Nijmegen Institute for International Health, Nijmegen, The Netherlands

Introduction

HIV-1 infection is more common in heterosexuals in Eastern and Southern Africa than in Europe and the US [1]. Within these countries HIV-1 infection usually has a higher prevalence in urban than in rural areas [1-6], as have other sexually transmitted diseases (STDs) [1,7]. A higher rate of heterosexual partner change in more affected areas could be an important determinant of this increased prevalence [1]. Extensive quantitative information on sexual partner change and condom use has recently been collected in Europe because of the HIV epidemic [8-10], but in Africa available information is still limited.

A cohort study of urban workers was initiated in a factory in Mwanza Municipality, Tanzania, in order to identify risk factors for HIV-1 seroconversion and for contracting other STDs. A second objective was to document changes in risk behaviour, in particular with respect to condom use and partner change after starting an intervention programme, and to determine whether these changes were associated with a reduced incidence of HIV-1 and other STDs.

In this paper quantitative results are reported at intake regarding sexual behaviour, in particular having multiple sexual partners and use of condoms. This intake took place from October 1991 to March 1992. The main aim of this analysis was to describe baseline information before interventions were undertaken at the factory, and to identify priorities for intervention. In a separate paper qualitative results are presented on the cultural and social background to the findings on sexual behaviour, risk perception, and behavioural change [11].

Methods

Study population

The study population comprised workers at a large urban factory with a work force of 1728 workers, 13% of whom were female. All workers were invited to enrol from the start of the study. A study clinic was created at the factory in addition to an existing clinic, as the latter was too small to cope with additional activities. Prior to starting the study, the willingness of the study population to participate was determined through an anonymous, self-administered questionnaire which produced a positive response of more than 90%. The study population has been advised that the aim of the study is to determine the health status of the workers, with special interest in sexually transmitted diseases and HIV-1 infection.

Pre- and post-HIV-test counselling was offered to all. Free treatment was provided to all study participants. Condoms were distributed free of charge by all staff present at the clinic. Where necessary, patients were referred to hospital for further investigation or treatment.

Data collection techniques

All respondents were interviewed in a private room for 30 to 45 minutes in Kiswahili by trained interviewers, using a structured and pre-coded questionnaire which was slightly different for men and women. The questionnaire covered demographic and socio-economic variables, health and sexually transmitted diseases, sexual partners and condom use, and finally sexual techniques. For the construction of the questionnaire, use was made of information from qualitative research both within the same Region and elsewhere in Tanzania.

Through pre-testing a number of modifications were made, both in the ordering of questions and in the content. In particular questions on sexual techniques other than vaginal sexual intercourse were found to cause embarrassment. Questions on oral-genital sexual contact were omitted, and questions on anal intercourse and masturbation put at the end of the questionnaire. Questions on types of sexual partners, frequency of sexual contact, and use of condoms proved to be less sensitive.

In the questionnaire a distinction was made between four types of partners: (1) spouse, (2) a partner one lives with but is not married to, (3) a steady partner one is not married to and does not live with, and (4) a casual partner. The last was defined by one respondent as "a strange face with whom who have sex once and then forget" [11]; in the questionnaire a casual partner was defined as any sexual partner not considered by respondent to be a steady partner. For further information on these different types of partners we refer to Nnko et al. [11]. As fewer than 1% of respondents reported having a partner in group (2), this type of partner has been considered as spouse in the analysis. Group (3) will be referred to in this paper as steady partner. After the interview respondents were physically examined, counselled, and bled for serological testing.

Data analysis
Data were analysed separately for males and females. Interquartile range (IQR) has been used as a measure of dispersion for skewed distributions. Survival analysis was used to determine the age of starting sexual intercourse, age at marriage, and the duration of marriage. Comparisons between survival curves were tested for statistical significance with the log rank test [12]. Stepwise logistic regression was used to simultaneously adjust for various variables of interest. Variables were eligible for inclusion in the regression model if they were a priori thought to be of interest (for example age) or showed an association with sexual partner change or condom use on univariate analysis. In order to assess the repeatability of responses, repeat questionnaires were administered on a sub-sample. In addition, a comparison was made with responses obtained from unstructured or semi-structured interviews by social scientists. For most variables a good repeatability could be demonstrated (kappa>0.80). However, for some variables such as religion repeatability was only moderate (0.5<kappa<0.8), perhaps because changing churches is not uncommon. For information on casual partners repeatability was good for contacts less than a month ago, but only moderate for contacts more than a month ago.

Results

In the first 19 weeks of the study 1096 workers (926 male, 170 female) were enrolled, comprising 62% of the male and 76% of the female work force. In comparison with the data on all factory workers, study participants were more likely to be aged below 25 years (18% vs 10%).

Age at first sexual intercourse and at first marriage
The age distribution at first sexual intercourse is presented in Fig. 1 for men and Fig.2 for women. By the 15th birthday 16% of male and 6% of female respondents reported having had sexual intercourse; by the 17th birthday these percentages were 44% and 33% respectively. By the 19th and 21st birthday 75% and 91% of men and women reported having had sexual intercourse respectively. Little difference was observed between men and women (log rank test $\chi_1 2$ 1.4, $P>0.2$). Secular changes in the age at first sexual intercourse were not observed.

The cumulative age distribution at first and consecutive marriages is also presented in Figs. 1 and 2. By their 21st birthdays 21% of men and 46% of women had married. Women have their first marriage at a younger age than men (log rank test $\chi_1 2$ 17.9, $P<0.0001$). Overall, 0.2% of men and 23.5% of women in this study population had not yet married by the age of 40 years.

In those who had ever married, the median period of having had premarital sexual intercourse (that is the difference between the age at first marriage and the age at first sexual intercourse) was 5 years (IQR 2 to 10 years) in men and 1 year (IQR 0 to 2.5 years) in women.

Second and third marriages were more common among men than women (Figures 1 and 2). By their 45th birthday 52% of men and 31% of women had married for a second time. By their 55th birthday, 33% of men and 7% of women had married for a third time. For women all second and third marriages took place after previous marriages had ended. Men had no spouse from an earlier marriage at the time of their second and third marriage in 223/280 (80%) and 53/70 (76%) of these marriages respectively.

Stability of marriage
The probability for a marriage to end (by divorce or death of the partner) was estimated to be 19% after 5 years of marriage for male workers and 22% for female workers. After 10 years 30% of marriages of male workers and 39% of marriages of female workers have ended. Marriage survival was significantly higher for men than for women (log rank $\chi_1 2=3.9$, $P<0.05$). The survival curves were similar for first and second marriages (log rank $\chi_1 2=0.6$, $P>0.25$).

Marital, steady, and casual partners
At the time of interview 724/926 (78%) of the male and 76/170 (45%) of the female factory workers were married and living together with their spouse. Of the 724 married men 45 (6%) had two wives, the others had one wife only. Among the married respondents 607/717 (85%) of the men and 71/76 (93%) of the women reported having

Figure 1. Cumulative percentage by age of having first sexual intercourse and first, second, third, and fourth marriage in 926 male factory workers

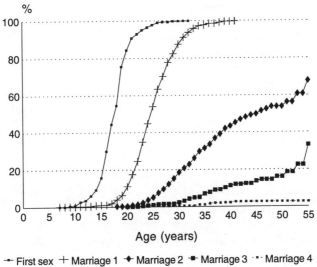

— First sex   + Marriage 1   ◆ Marriage 2   ▪ Marriage 3   ·· Marriage 4

Figure 2. Cumulative percentage by age of having first sexual intercourse and first, second and third marriage in 170 female factory workers

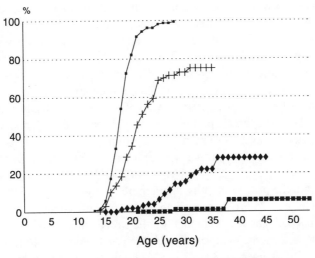

— First sex   + Marriage 1   ◆ Marriage 2   ▪ Marriage 3

Table 1. Distribution of having various types of partners in 926 male and 170 female urban factory workers

| | Number(%) | | |
| | Steady partner* (one or more) with whom sexual intercourse took place in past month | Casual partner** within | |
		past 4 weeks	past 12 months
Males			
Married	147/ 724 (20%)	44/ 724 (6%)	150/ 724 (21%)
Single	61/ 149 (41%)	29/ 149 (19%)	81/ 149 (54%)
Married but living apart, separated or widowed	20/ 53 (38%)	5/ 53 (9%)	22/ 53 (42%)
Females			
Married	6/ 76 (7%)	0/ 76 (0%)	5/ 76 (5%)
Single	27/ 61 (45%)	1/ 61 (2%)	8/ 61 (13%)
Married but living apart, separated or widowed	10/ 33 (29%)	1/ 33 (3%)	5/ 33 (14%)

* A steady partner is defined as a sexual partner other than a spouse one has a relationship with for some length of time.
** A casual partner is any sexual partner who is not a spouse or steady partner.

had sex with their spouse in the past four weeks (men: median 4 times, IQR 2 to 8; women: median 5, IQR 2 to 9).

Having one or more (non-marital) steady partners was reported by 294/926 (32%) of men and 75/170 (44%) of women, and was more common among those not currently married (Table 1). Among the respondents with one or more steady partners 228/294 (78%) of the men and 43/75 (57%) of the women reported having had sex with their steady partner in the past 4 weeks (men: median 3 times, IQR 2 to 5; women: median 1, IQR 1 to 2). The median duration of reported current steady partnerships was 7 months (IQR 4–18 months) for men and 24 months (IQR 12–36 months) for women. Men were usually older than their female steady partner. Men of all ages had steady partners, while 351/364 (96%) of their female partners were aged less than 35 years. The male steady partners reported by women were in all age groups.

Having ever had a casual sexual partner was reported by 654/926 (71%) of men and 63/170 (37%) of women. 253/925 (27%) of men and 18/170 (11%) of women had had a casual partner within the past 12 months, again more commonly among those not currently married. Only 15/253 (6%) of men and 1/18 (6%) of women stated they met the casual partner in a bar. The rest were met 'on the street' (men 167/253 [66%], women 5/18 [26%]), at a friend's house (men 24/253 [9%], women 5/18 [28%]), or at a party (men 13/253 [5%], women 2/18 [11%]). Other, less frequent possibilities included wedding or burial ceremonies and discos. More information on meeting places with casual partners is given by Nnko et al [11].

Table 2. Determinants for having had more than one sexual partner in the past month in 926 male urban factory workers

Risk factor	Number with 2+ sexual partners/ Nr seen (%)	χ^2 test	Odds ratio (95% CI) Crude	Adjusted for significant factors
Age		P>0.05		
15-24	25/ 146 (17)		I	I
25-34	77/ 297 (26)		1.7 (1.0-2.8)	1.3 (0.7-2.6)
35-44	75/ 350 (21)		1.3 (0.8-2.2)	0.4 (0.2-0.9)
45+	28/ 133 (21)		1.3 (0.7-2.3)	0.8 (0.4-0.7)
Residence		P>0.05		
Mwanza Municipality	175/ 826 (21)		I	I
Outside Municipality	28/ 94 (30)		1.6 (1.0-2.5)	1.1 (0.6-1.7)
Birth place		P<0.001		
Mwanza Region	153/ 557 (27)		I	I
Shinyanga/ Mara	37/ 164 (23)		0.8 (0.5-1.2)	0.7 (0.5-1.1)
Kagera	3/ 39 (8)		0.2 (0.1-0.7)	0.4 (0.1-1.2)
Other	12/ 166 (7)		0.2 (0.1-0.4)	0.2 (0.1-0.5)
Marital status		P<0.01		
Married	179/ 724 (25)		I	I
Never married	22/ 149 (15)		0.5 (0.3-0.9)	0.6 (0.3-1.3)
Married but living apart, separated or widowed	4/ 53 (8)		0.2 (0.1-0.7)	0.3 (0.1-0.8)
Education				
<5 yr primary	24/ 88 (27)	P=0.01	1.2 (0.7-2.0)	1.1 (0.6-1.8)
5-7 yr primary	168/ 717	trend:	I	I
secondary education	13/ 121 (11)	P<0.01	0.4 (0.2-0.7)	0.5 (0.3-1.0)
Income per capita				
<1500	57/ 186 (31)	P<0.001	I	I
1500	43/ 176 (24)	trend:	0.7 (0.5-1.2)	0.7 (0.4-1.2)
2000	43/ 168 (26)	P<0.001	0.8 (0.5-1.2)	0.8 (0.5-1.4)
2500	31/ 152 (20)		0.6 (0.4-1.0)	0.7 (0.4-1.2)
3500	30/ 239 (13)		0.3 (0.2-0.5)	0.5 (0.3-0.8)

* Factors adjusted for in logistic regression were age, birthplace, marital status, education, and income per capita.
** (monthly household income in Tanzania Shillings)/(number of adults + 1/2 number of children)

Determinants of having multiple partners in men
Having had more than one sexual partner (including the spouse where applicable) in the past month was reported by 205/926 (22%) of men and 8/170 (5%) of women. Determinants of having multiple sexual partners among men are presented in Table 2. The group of women was too small for such detailed analysis.

Table 3. Condom use ever and condom use last month by risk factor in 926 male urban factory workers

Risk factor	Condom use ever			Condom use last month		
	Nr using/ Total (%)	Crude OR (P-value)	OR (95% CI) adjusted for significant factors[1]	Nr using/ Total (%)	Crude OR (P-value)	OR (95% CI) adjusted for significant factors[2]
Age						
15-24	46/ 145 (32)	I (P<0.001)	I	9/ 145 (6)	I P<0.05)	
25-34	48/ 297 (16)	0.4	0.5 (0.3-0.9)	9/ 296 (3)	0.5	
35-44	40/ 349 (11)	0.3	0.4 (0.3-0.8) }	10/ 483 (2)	0.3	
45+	7/ 133 (5)	0.1	0.3 (0.1-0.7) }			
Residence						
Municipality	135/ 824 (16)	I (P>0.05)	I	27/ 824 (3)	I (P>0.05)	
Outside Municipality	4/ 94 (4)	0.2	0.3 (0.1-1.0)	1/ 94 (1)	0.3	
Having had sex with casual partner						
past month	25/ 78 (32)	3.8	3.5 (1.9-6.4)	11/ 77 (14)	13.4	13.1(4.8-35.8)
1-4 months	34/ 111 (31)	3.6	3.2 (1.9-5.4)	7/ 111 (6)	5.5	5.7 (1.9-17.0)
> 4 months ago or never	81/ 734 (11)	I P<0.001)	I	9/ 735 (1)	I P<0.001)	I
Having had sex with steady partner past month						
Yes	49/ 227 (22)	1.8	2.1 (1.3-3.3)	15/ 227 (7)	3.7	5.9 (2.4-14.6)
No	92/ 697 (13)	I P<0.001)	I	13/ 697 (2)	I P<0.001)	I
Education						
<5 year	2/ 87 (2)	0.2	0.2 (0.0-1.2) }			
5-7 year	96/ 716 (13)	I (P<0.001)	I }	18/ 803 (2)	I P<0.001)	I
secondary	43/ 121 (36)	3.6	3.5 (2.2-5.8)	10/ 121 (8)	3.9	4.4 (1.8-10.8)
		(trend:P<0.001)			(trend:P<0.01)	
Income per capita						
<1500	19/ 185 (10)	I (P<0.001)	I	5/ 186 (3)	I (P>0.05)	
1500	14/ 176 (8)	0.8	0.9 (0.4-2.0)	2/ 175 (1)	0.4	
2000	16/ 168 (10)	0.9	1.0 (0.5-2.2)	4/ 168 (2)	0.9	
2500	29/ 151 (19)	2.1	2.1 (1.1-4.3)	6/ 151 (4)	1.5	
3500	61/ 239 (26)	3.0	1.8 (1.0-3.5)	11/ 239 (5)	1.7	
		(trend:P<0.001)				
Circumcision						
Yes	88/ 429 (21)	2.2	1.7 (1.1-2.5)	16/ 431 (4)	1.5	
No	53/ 495 (11)	I (P<0.001)	I	12/ 493 (2)	I (P>0.05)	

Table 3, continued

Risk factor	Condom use ever			Condom use last month		
	Nr using/ Total (%)	Crude OR (P-value)	OR (95% CI) adjusted for significant factors[1]	Nr using/ Total (%)	Crude OR (P-value)	OR (95% CI) adjusted for significant factors[2]
Genital discharge last						
Never	67/ 509 (13)	I (P<0.01)		14/ 510 (3)	I (P<0.05)	I
4 months +	57/ 364 (16)	1.2		9/ 363 (2)	0.9	0.5 (0.2-1.4)
<4 months/ now	17/ 51 (33)	3.3		5/ 51 (10)	3.9	3.7 (1.1-12.2)
		(trend: P<0.01)			(trend: P<0.0005)	
Birth place						
Mwanza Region	62/ 556 (11)	I (P=0.001)		13/ 556 (2)	I (P<0.01)	I
Shinyanga/	31/ 164 (19)	1.7		5/ 163 (3)	1.3	1.1 (0.3-3.5)
Mara	12/ 39 (31)	3.5		5/ 39 (13)	6.1	6.7 (1.7-25.6)
Kagera	36/ 165 (22)	2.2		5/ 166 (3)	1.3	1.6 (0.5-5.3)
Other						
Marital status						
Married	5/ 723 (12)	I (P<0.01)		14/ 722 (2)	I (P<0.05)	
Single	49/ 148 (33)	3.7		11/ 149 (7)	4.0	
Married but living apart, separated or widowed	7/ 53 (13)	1.1		3/ 53 (6)	3.0	

I Significant factors adjusted for in logistic regression were age, residence, education, income, circumcision, having had sex with a steady partner, and having had sex with a casual partner

2 Significant factors adjusted for in logistic regression were birthplace, education, having had sex with a steady partner, and having had sex with a casual partner

3 (monthly household income in Tanzania Shilling)/(number of adults + 1/ 2 number of children)

Having more than one sexual partner was reported by 179/724 (25%) of married men, 22/149 (13%) of single men, and 4/53 (8%) of those who were married but living apart, or were separated or widowed (Table 2). Of the 179 married men with more than one sexual partner only 33 (18%) had had sex with more than one spouse; the other 82% had had extramarital relationships. Factors associated with having had multiple sexual partners in the past month (after adjusting for the other significant variables in logistic regression) were: being born in Mwanza or the neighbouring Mara or Shinyanga Regions, having had less education or having a low income, and being married. Having had more than one sexual partner in the past month was also associated with having ever had a genital discharge. This was not included in the regression model as it was thought to be a consequence rather than a determinant of sexual partner change.

Determinants of condom use in men
Overall, 141/924 (15%) of men and 30/170 (18%) of women had ever used a condom. Only 28/924 (3%) of men and 5/170 (3%) of women had used a condom in the past month. A number of determinants of condom use in men were identified (Table 3). The group of women was too small for this analysis.

Factors associated with condom use in men after adjusting for the other significant variables in logistic regression were being in the younger age groups, living within the municipality, having had sexual intercourse with a casual or steady partner, having a higher level of education, having a higher income, having had a recent genital discharge, being circumcised, and being born in Kagera (a neighbouring Region with a high prevalence of HIV-1 infection). Condoms were used most frequently with casual partners (18% of sexual contacts), much less with steady partners (2%), and hardly with spouses (0.2%).

Neither sexual partner change, nor condom use were found to be associated with the religion of respondents.

Discussion

This study shows that high risk behaviour in this group of factory workers was widespread, in particular among men; 22% of male workers reported having had more than one sexual partner in the past month, 97% had not used a condom at all in the past month, and 85% reported they had never used them in their life.

It is difficult to assess the validity of self-reported sexual behaviour. Age at first sexual intercourse may have been misreported due to recall bias, or because of a tendency to give socially desirable answers. The direction of the latter bias is likely to have been towards higher ages at first sexual intercourse, in particular among women. If this bias has occurred, the period of premarital sexual intercourse will have been underestimated.

During pre-testing, people reported to be at ease answering questions on partner relations (but not questions on sexual techniques). Having had multiple partners in the past month was reported by a large proportion of men (22%), but less so by women (5%). In men it was associated with having a genital discharge or genital ulcer at physical examination (unpublished data), suggesting that this high risk behaviour is reported with some accuracy. As women are not socially expected to have many sexual partners, in particular not when they are married, this may have biased (i.e. reduced) the number of sexual partners reported by women.

Further validation studies are needed. Validation of self-reported sexual behaviour has been attempted in various studies aiming at quantifying risk behaviour for STDs and HIV, with encouraging results [13-18]. However, very few such studies appear to have been carried out in Africa, and much more work on this issue is needed [19].

A limitation of the study is self-selection bias, as 37% of workers had not (yet) enrolled at the time of this analysis. The direction of this analysis is uncertain: those declining to participate might have had increased risk behaviour (and be afraid to be tested for HIV-1 and other sexually transmitted diseases) or reduced risk behaviour (and have less interest in being tested for sexually transmitted diseases).

Age at first sexual intercourse in this study is similar to that reported from other countries in Africa [20–22], Haiti [23], and Europe [8,10,24], starting in the mid-teens in both sexes, and with a period of premarital sexual intercourse of several years in most men and a substantial proportion of women. Contrary to findings in Europe [9], no evidence was found for a shift over time towards younger ages for first sexual intercourse. IEC on sexual relationships and condom use should therefore start before the mid-teens and preferably include education at primary schools.

Rates of acquisition of marital partners and marital breakdown appear to be small in comparison with the rates of acquisition and breakdown of steady and casual partnerships. Polygamy only plays a minor role in sexual partner change in this population. Follow-up is expected to provide more information on the relative contribution of marital partner change to overall partner change. Female factory workers were less likely to get married, and after marriage were more likely to divorce than male workers. Female factory workers appear to be a special group, and are probably not representative for the general female population.

Although extramarital relationships were reported much more commonly than for instance in the UK [8], similar rates of having extramarital sexual partners have been reported from Uganda [25], Zaire [20,26], Zimbabwe [27], Ghana [21], and other countries in Africa [22].

Many more men had sexual intercourse in the past month with steady than with casual partners (although over the past year these proportions did not differ). As relationships with steady partners usually last less than two years, steady partnerships may contribute substantially to the overall rate of sexual partner change and therefore to the risk of acquiring HIV or others sexually transmitted diseases. This implies that condom promotion needs to be expanded beyond groups such as commercial sex workers and their clients.

No association was found between age group and having multiple partners, contrary to findings in Europe, where having multiple partners was more frequently reported by young adults [9,10]. However, the types of partner vary with age, casual and steady partners becoming less common and spouses more common with increasing age (data not shown). Having had multiple partners in the past month was more often reported by men with less education and a low income. This is in contrast to previous reports from African countries [22], where a higher level of education was associated with more often having had casual partners in the past 12 months. Perhaps behaviour has changed in those with more education, although response bias can not easily be ruled out: respondents with more education might have been more receptive to health education and have answered questions accordingly, without necessarily having changed behaviour. HIV-1 infection was not associated with level of education or income (data not shown). This is consistent with a higher risk in the past and a lower risk at present for better educated men.

Only 3% of male and female respondents had used a condom in the past month. Condoms were used mostly with casual partners, much less with steady partners, and least of all with spouses. However, even with casual partners, condoms protected only 18% of the sexual contacts which took place in the past month. This low use of condoms was not unexpected [6,28,29]. However, the data suggest that condom use has increased recently: condoms were used more by the young, better educated, and those having been born in high risk Regions. The increased condom use by the young and better educated has also been described in The Gambia [30]. The increased condom use in those with higher incomes may have been partly due to fewer economic barriers to condom use for this group. Unfortunately, groups with low education and income were not only more likely to report having had multiple sexual partners, but also less likely to report having used condoms. This group should be a priority for intervention.

Acknowledgements

We thank the Principal Secretary, Ministry of Health and the Director General, National Institute for Medical Research for permission to carry out the study and to publish its results. We thank Dr G Lwihula and Prof R A Coutinho for support in developing the questionnaires and Prof A S Muller, and Dr C M Varkevisser for critically reviewing the manuscript. The research for this publication was financed by the Netherlands' Minister for Development Cooperation, Section for Research and Technology, P.O.Box 20061, 2500 EB, The Hague, as part of the Tanzania-Netherlands Research Project on AIDS and HIV Infection in Mwanza Region. Responsibility for the contents and for the opinions expressed rests solely with the authors; publication does not constitute an endorsement by the Netherlands' Minister for Development Co-operation.

References

1. Piot P, Laga M, Ryder R, et al. The global epidemiology of HIV infection: continuity, heterogeneity, and change. J AIDS 1990;3:403-412.
2. Piot P, Plummer FA, Mhalu FS, Lamboray JL, Chin J, Mann JM. AIDS: an international perspective. Science 1988;239:573-579.
3. Rwandan HIV seroprevalence study group. Nationwide community-based serological survey of HIV-1 and other human retrovirus infections in a Central African country. Lancet 1989;i:941-943.
4. Killewo J, Nyamuryekung'e K, Sandström A, et al. Prevalence of HIV-1 infection in the Kagera region of Tanzania: a population-based study. AIDS 1990;4:1081-1085.
5. Serwadda D, Wawer MJ, Musgrave SD, Sewankambo NK, Kaplan JE, Gray RH. HIV risk factors in three geographic strata of rural Rakai District, Uganda. AIDS 1992;6:983-989.
6. Barongo LR, Borgdorff MW, Mosha FF, et al. The epidemiology of HIV-1 infection in urban areas, roadside settlements and rural villages in Mwanza Region, Tanzania. AIDS 1992;6:1521-1528.
7. Laga M, Nzila N, Goeman J. The interrelationship of sexually transmitted diseases and HIV infection: implications for the control of both epidemics in Africa. AIDS 1991;5(suppl 1):S55-S63.
8. Johnson AM, Wadsworth J, Elliott P, et al. A pilot study of sexual lifestyle in a random sample of the population of Great Britain. AIDS 1989;3:135-141.
9. Johnson AM, Wadsworth J, Wellings K, Bradshaw S, Field J. Sexual lifestyles and HIV risk. Nature 1992;360:410-412.
10. ACSF investigators. AIDS and sexual behaviour in France. Nature 1992;360:407-409.

11. Nnko S, Mwanga J, Varkevisser C, et al. Risk perception and behavioural change in relation to AIDS – An exploratory study among factory workers in Mwanza town, Tanzania. In: Dautzenberg M, Nnko S, Chiduo B et al. Action research for the development of interventions to reduce HIV transmission in Mwanza Region, Tanzania. Amsterdam: KIT Press (in press)

12. Armitage P, Berry G. Statistical methods in medical research. 2nd Ed. Oxford: Blackwell Scientific Publications, 1987:429-433.

13. McQueen D. Understanding sexual behaviour. AIDS 1992;6:329-330.

14. Coates RA, Calzavara LM, Soskolne CL, et al. Validity of sexual histories in a prospective study of male sexual contacts of men with AIDS or an AIDS related condition. Am J Epidemiol 1988;128:719-728.

15. James NJ, Bignell CJ, Gillies PA. The reliability of self-reported sexual behaviour. AIDS 1991;5:333-336.

16. Upchurch DM, Weisman CS, Shepherd M, et al. Interpartner reliability of reporting of recent sexual behaviors. Am J Epidemiol 1991;134:1159-1166.

17. Seage GR, Mayer KH, Horsburgh CR, Cai B, Lamb GA. Corroboration of sexual histories among male homosexual couples. Am J Epidemiol 1992;135:79-84.

18. Wilson D, Chiroro P, Lavelle S, Mutero C. Sex workers, client sex behaviour and condom use in Harare, Zimbabwe. AIDS Care 1989;1:269-280.

19. Pickering H. Asking questions on sexual behaviour ... testing methods from the social sciences. Health Pol Plann 1988;3:237-244.

20. Bertrand JT, Makani B, Hassig SE, et al. AIDS-related knowledge, sexual behaviour, and condom use among men and women in Kinshasa, Zaire. Am J Public Health 1991;81:53-58.

21. Neequaye AR, Neequaye JE, Biggar RJ. Factors that could influence the spread of AIDS in Ghana, West Africa: knowledge of AIDS, sexual behavior, prostitution, and traditional medical practices. J Acq Imm Def Syndr 1991;4:914-919.

22. Carael M, Cleland J, Adeokun L, and Collaborating Investigators. Overview and selected findings of sexual behaviour surveys. AIDS 1991;5(Suppl):S65-S75.

23. Halsey NA, Coberly JS, Holt E, et al. Sexual behaviour, smoking, and HIV-1 infection in Haitian women. JAMA 1992;267:2062-2066.

24. Forman D, Chivers C. Sexual behaviour of young and middle aged men in England and Wales. Br Med J 1989;298:1137-1142.

25. Müller O, Barugahare L, Schwartländer B, et al. HIV prevalence, attitudes and behaviour in clients of a confidential HIV testing and counselling centre in Uganda. AIDS 1992;6:869-874.

26. Ryder RW, Ndilu M, Hassig SE, et al. Heterosexual transmission of HIV-1 among employees and their spouses at two large businesses in Zaire. AIDS 1990;4:725-732.

27. Bassett MT, Latif AS, Katzenstein DA, Emmanuel JC. Sexual behaviour and risk factors for HIV infection in a group of male factory workers who donated blood in Harare, Zimbabwe. J Acq Imm Def Syndr 1992;5:556-559.

28. Goldberg HI, Lee NC, Oberie MW, Peterson HB. Knowledge about condoms and their use in less developed countries during a period of rising AIDS prevalence. Bull Wrld Hlth Org 1989;67:85-91.

29. Forster SJ, Furley KE. 1988 public awareness survey on AIDS and condoms in Uganda. AIDS 1989;3:147-154.

30. Wilkins HA, Alonso P, Baldeh S, et al. Knowledge of AIDS, use of condoms and results of counselling subjects with asymptomatic HIV2 infection in The Gambia. AIDS Care 1989;1:247-256.

9

HIV-1 incidence and HIV-1 associated mortality and morbidity in a cohort of urban factory workers in Tanzania

Martien W Borgdorff[1,4]*, Longin R Barongo*[1]*, Arnoud H Klokke*[2]*, John Changalucha*[1]*,*
James N Newell[1,3,6]*, Kesheni P Senkoro*[1]*, Johan P Velema*[5]*, RM Gabone*[1]

Submitted for publication

Summary

Objective. To determine HIV-1 incidence and HIV-1 associated mortality and morbidity in a prospective cohort study.

Methods. The study population was a cohort of 1,772 urban factory workers in northwest Tanzania. The study took place from October 1991 to September 1993. Outcome measures were HIV-1 seroconversion, death, clinical diagnoses by assistant medical officers and laboratory diagnoses in the field laboratory. HIV-1 infection was determined by ELISA and Western Blot.

Results. HIV-1 incidence was 1.2 (95% CI 0.7–1.8) per 100 person-years (pyr). Crude annual mortality was 4.9 per 100 pyr in those with and 0.3 in those without HIV-1 infection, giving an age and sex adjusted mortality ratio of 12.9 (95% CI 5.4–30.7). Of all deaths, 62% were attributable to HIV-1 infection. Clinical diagnoses in men associated with HIV-1 infection included fever, bacterial skin infections, tonsillitis/sore throat, diarrhoea, and dysentery. HIV-1 infection in men was also associated with the prevalence and incidence of low body mass index, and with the presence and level of malaria parasitaemia, with anaemia, with *E histolytica, G intestinalis, T hominis* and *S stercoralis* infection, and gonorrhoea. In women diarrhoea, herpes zoster, and genital discharge were associated with HIV-1 infection.

Conclusion. HIV-1 was the major cause of death and substantially contributed to an increased morbidity in this adult population with an HIV-1 prevalence of 12% and an HIV-1 incidence of 1.2%. The number of HIV-1 seroconversions was only slightly larger than that of HIV-1 associated deaths, suggesting that the HIV-1 epidemic may have reached a steady state in this population.

1 National Institute for Medical Research, Mwanza, Tanzania
2 Bugando Medical Centre, Mwanza
3 AMREF, Mwanza
4 Royal Tropical Institute, Amsterdam, The Netherlands
5 Nijmegen Institute of International Health, Nijmegen, The Netherlands
6 London School of Hygiene and Tropical Medicine, UK

Introduction

When studies are planned to evaluate the efficacy of interventions to reduce HIV-1 transmission for instance through condom promotion or STD control, and in future through immunization against HIV-1, a reasonable estimate of the incidence of HIV-1 infection is required for sample size determination [1]. However, published literature on the incidence of HIV-1 infection in Africa appears to be limited [2], probably because incidence can only be measured in longitudinal studies which are difficult and costly to perform [3].

HIV-1 infection has been shown to contribute substantially to mortality in hospitals in Africa [4–10]. An obvious limitation of these studies is their selection bias, as in Africa many people die at home. Evidence from community based studies is starting to emerge as well: in Rwanda and Uganda HIV-1 associated mortality was shown to be substantial [11,12]. Quantification of HIV-1-associated mortality is important for assessment and prediction of the demographic and socioeconomic impact of the epidemic [13,14].

Information concerning the clinical spectrum of HIV-1 infection in Africa is critical to the formulation of treatment and prophylactic regimens and may contribute to diagnostic algorithms [15]. So far, the clinical manifestations of HIV-1 infection in Africa have mainly been studied in cross-sectional studies among hospitalized patients in large referral hospitals and very little information is available from community-based prospective studies [15].

A cohort study among urban factory workers in Mwanza, Tanzania, was started in October 1991 in order to determine the incidence of and risk factors for HIV-1 infection and other STDs, describe changes in sexual high risk behaviour following an intervention, and describe the natural history of HIV-1 infection. The prevalence of and risk factors for HIV-1 infection at intake of the cohort were found to be similar to those in the general urban population [16,17].

In this paper we describe the HIV-1 incidence and HIV-1 associated mortality and morbidity in this cohort from October 1991 to September 1993.

Methods

Study population
The study population comprised workers at a large urban factory with a work force of 2,038 workers (1,706 men, 332 women). Enrolment started in October 1991 and continued throughout, both for new employees and those initially declining to participate. A study clinic was created at the factory to supplement an existing clinic, as the latter was too small to cope with additional activities. The study population has been advised that the aim of the study is to determine the health status of the workers, with special interest in sexually transmitted diseases and HIV-1 infection and has been invited to present themselves for registration at the study clinic. The data presented here cover a study period of two years, from 1 October 1991 to 30 September 1993.

Data collection techniques

All respondents were interviewed, physically examined and underwent laboratory investigations at intake and at four-monthly intervals thereafter. Free medical treatment was provided to all study participants at intake, follow-up visits, and any time they presented in between. Where necessary, patients were referred to hospital for further investigation or treatment.

In the study clinic laboratory 10 ml of venous blood was taken using a vacuum system at intake and at the four-monthly follow-up visits. Serological testing for HIV-1 antibodies took place with the Vironostika anti-HTLV-III ELISA (Organon, Boxtel, The Netherlands). All non-negative samples were tested with Western Blot (Organon, Epitope, Beaverton, Oregon, USA). The Western Blot was considered positive if at least two of the gp41, gp120, and gp160 bands were present [18]. Pre- and post-HIV-1-test counselling was offered to all. After pre-test counselling a separate blood sample was taken for HIV-1 testing from those wishing to know their HIV-1 test result. The HIV-1 results were made known to the counsellor and through the counsellor to the individual concerned only. Other staff at the factory clinic were blind to the HIV-1 status of individuals.

Deaths among study participants were identified by a follow-up worker tracing non-attenders and through the welfare officer at the factory responsible for paying an allowance to the relatives of the deceased. The latter officer knew of all deaths identified, suggesting that his registration of deaths was comprehensive. The household of the deceased was visited two to six months after death in order to identify the cause of death, using open-ended questions, a structured questionnaire, and a death notification form if available. For those who died in hospital, hospital records were traced in order to get the hospital diagnosis. The cause of death was determined from hospital records if available and otherwise by consensus of a group of three medical officers, including one specialist in internal medicine, blinded to HIV-1 status of the deceased.

Clinical diagnoses, largely based on history taking and examination, were made and recorded by an assistant medical officer and coded later by a medical officer. Diagnoses based on laboratory results (e.g. malaria or gonorrhoea) were coded under the relevant syndrome (e.g. fever or genital discharge) as a clinical diagnosis, while results of the field laboratory were analyzed directly. From April 1992 a balance scale was used for routine determination of body weight. Previous weight measurements were excluded from analysis. On request of the assistant medical officer the following laboratory tests could be carried out: urine albumen, glucose, and sediment, stools smear, smear for gram stain from genital discharge, and blood smear for determining malaria parasitaemia. Routine determination of haemoglobin levels was introduced in May 1992. All laboratory tests were carried out according to standardized procedures and results were recorded on a pre-coded form.

Data analysis

Events (deaths, cases of disease) were included if they occurred inside the defined follow-up period. Three sets of person-years of follow-up were calculated. For HIV-1 incidence follow-up included the time period between the first and last negative HIV-1 test result plus for seroconverters half the time period between the last negative and

Table 1. Incidence of HIV-1 infection in a cohort of 1567 non-HIV-1 infected urban factory workers

Age group (years)	Number enroled (HIV-)	Number of sero-conversions	Person-years (pyr) of follow-up	Incidence/ 100 pyr (95%CI)
Males				
15-25	340	1	211.7	0.5 (0.0-2.6)
25-34	409	5	342.8	1.5 (0.5-3.4)
35-44	411	7	433.1	1.6 (0.7-3.3)
45+	165	2	183.3	1.1 (0.1-3.9)
All males	1325	15	1171.0	1.3 (0.7-2.1)
Females				
15-25	105	0	64.7	0.0 (0.0-5.5)
25-34	97	2	84.2	2.4 (0.3-8.3)
35-44	31	0	38.0	0.0 (0.0-9.3)
45+	9	0	8.0	0.0 (0.0-36.9)
All females	242	2	195.0	1.0 (0.1-3.7)
Total	1567	17	1365.9	1.2 (0.7-2.0)

first positive HIV-1 result. For *mortality* the follow-up period included the time from the first HIV-1 result until the end of follow-up; the end of follow-up was defined as the date of: (1) death or leaving the factory, (2) one year after the last HIV-1 result or (3) 30 September 1993, whichever came first.

For *morbidity* the follow-up period included the time from two weeks after the first HIV-1 result to two weeks after the last. The period of two weeks was arbitrarily selected to ensure that diagnoses at intake were excluded. Follow-up was calculated separately for those with and without HIV-1 infection; in seroconverters, the time between the last negative and first positive HIV-1 result was excluded.

It was assumed that incidence rates had a Poisson distribution both for calculating confidence intervals and for testing differences between rates. The population attributable risk was calculated as the difference of the mortality rate in the total population and the mortality rate in those without HIV-1 infection and the population etiological fraction as the ratio of the population excess rate and the mortality rate in the total population. In the analysis of HIV-1 associated morbidity relative risk (RR) was defined as the ratio and attributable risk (AR) as the difference of the incidence rates in those with and without HIV-1 infection.

Results

Of the 2,038 factory workers 1,478/1,706 (87%) men and 294/332 (89%) women had enroled in the study. A total of 471 (27%) of these were lost to follow-up by the end of the study period. Defaulting was not associated with sex or HIV-1 infection (data not

Table 2. **Mortality rates in an urban factory in 205 workers with and 1567 workers without HIV-1 infection**

Age group (years)	HIV-1 infected				Non HIV-1 infected			
	Number*		Person-years of follow up	Mortality rate (/100 pyr)	Number*		Person-years of follow up	Mortality rate (/100 pyr)
	Enroled	Died			Enroled	Died		
Males								
15-25	17	0	21.2	0.0	340	1	421.8	0.2
25-34	71	3	100.8	3.0	409	0	561.8	0.0
35-44	54	9	78.8	11.4	411	2	629.2	0.3
45+	11	1	12.7	7.9	165	1	257.9	0.4
All males	153	13	213.6	6.1	1325	4	1870.7	0.2
Females								
15-25	14	0	17.8	0.0	105	0	132.1	0.0
25-34	26	0	35.1	0.0	97	3	131.1	2.3
35-44	11	1	17.0	5.9	31	0	51.1	0.0
45+	1	0	1.9	0.0	9	0	13.3	0.0
All females	52	1	71.9	1.4	242	3	327.5	0.9
Total	205	14	285.5	4.9	1567	7	2198.2	0.3

* HIV-1 status is given at enrolment. Seroconverters contribute person-years of follow-up to the groups without and with HIV-1 infection before and after seroconversion respectively.

shown), but was higher in those aged below 35 years (317/1,079=29%) than in those aged 35 years and over (154/693=22%)(χ^2 10.7; P<0.01).

At intake 153/1,478 (10.4%) men and 52/294 (17.7%) women were HIV-1 infected. In the study period 17 seroconversions took place in 1,365.9 person years of follow-up giving an HIV-1 incidence of 1.2 per 100 person-years of follow-up (95% CI 0.7–1.8). No association was found between seroconversion and age or sex; the power of the study to detect such associations was limited as the number of seroconversions was small (Table 1).

The crude annual mortality rate was 4.9 per 100 person-years in those with and 0.3 in those without HIV-1 infection (Table 2). The age and sex adjusted mortality ratio was 12.9 (95% CI 5.4–30.7). The population attributable risk was 0.5 per 100 person-years, and the population etiological fraction 62%.

Of the 14 HIV-1 infected people who died, one had cryptococcal meningitis, and the criteria of the WHO provisional clinical AIDS case definition [19] were met certainly by eight others and possibly by another two. The three without an AIDS diagnosis had pulmonary tuberculosis, diarrhoea, and pyomyositis respectively. Although because of data limitations the WHO clinical AIDS case definition could not be strictly applied, it seems likely that at least 3 out of 14 (21%) of HIV-1 infected people died before developing AIDS.

Table 3. The incidence of clinical diagnoses in a cohort of 1478 male factory workers

Clinical diagnosis	Number of cases		Incidence rate*		Relative risk	P-value**	Attributable risk (/100 pyr)
	HIV+	HIV-	HIV+	HIV-			
General							
Fever	219	1597	167.6	135.2	1.2	<0.01	32.4
Skin							
Scabies	17	94	13.0	8.0	1.6	ns	
Fungal skin infection	35	411	26.8	35.2	0.8	ns	
Bacterial skin infection	23	73	17.6	6.2	2.8	<0.0001	11.4
Herpes zoster	7	3	5.4	0.3	20.9	<0.0001	5.1
Herpes labialis	2	3	1.5	0.3	6.0	ns	
Allergic skin reaction	5	46	3.8	3.9	1.0	ns	
Skin ulcer	0	2	0.0	0.2	0.0	ns	
Skin other	2	25	1.5	2.1	0.7	ns	
Eyes/Neurological							
Conjunctivitis	39	363	29.8	31.1	1.0	ns	
Poor vision	1	7	0.8	0.6	1.3	ns	
Paraesthesia, neuropathy, neuritis, neuralgia	7	51	5.4	4.4	1.2	ns	
Headache	2	36	1.5	3.3	0.5	ns	
Anxiety/neurosis	3	16	2.3	1.4	1.7	ns	
Neurological other	2	20	1.5	1.7	0.9	ns	
Respiratory/ Ears							
Upper respiratory tract infection	61	542	46.7	46.4	1.0	ns	
Otitis media	9	43	6.9	3.7	1.9	ns	
Bronchial asthma	17	59	13.0	5.1	2.6	<0.001	79
Bronchitis	36	224	27.5	19.2	1.4	ns	
Resp tract infection unspecified	58	481	44.4	41.2	1.1	ns	
Lower resp. tract inf./ pneumonia	11	79	8.4	6.8	1.2	ns	
Respiratory other	14	64	10.7	5.5	2.0	<0.05	5.2
Circulatory							
Hypertension	0	57	0.0	4.9	0.0	<0.05	-4.9
Lymphadenitis	5	15	3.8	1.3	3.0	ns	
Circulatory other	0	3	0.0	0.3	0.0	ns	

Table 3, continued

Clinical diagnosis	Number of cases		Incidence rate*		Relative risk	P-value**	Attribut-able risk (/100 pyr)
	HIV+	HIV-	HIV+	HIV-			
Gastrointestinal							
Stomatitis	6	70	4.6	6.0	0.8	ns	
Sore throat/tonsillitis	47	233	36.0	19.9	1.8	<0.001	16.1
Gastritis/dyspepsia	30	302	23.0	25.9	0.9	ns	
Diarrhoea	64	364	49.0	31.2	1.6	<0.01	17.8
Dysentery	56	256	42.9	21.9	2.0	<0.0001	21.0
Piles/haemorrhoids	2	13	1.5	1.1	1.4	ns	
Gastrointestinal other	28	176	21.4	15.1	1.4	ns	
Urogenital							
Urinary tract infection	42	300	32.1	25.7	1.3	ns	
Urethral discharge	19	90	14.5	7.7	1.9	<0.05	6.8
Orchitis/epididimitis	9	16	6.9	1.4	5.0	<0.0001	5.5
Genital ulcer	4	21	3.1	1.8	1.7	ns	
Urogenital other	3	14	2.3	1.2	1.9	ns	
Extremities							
Arthritis/arthalgia	13	46	9.9	3.9	2.5	<0.01	6.0
Low backache	20	214	15.3	18.3	0.8	na	
Trauma/injury/wounds	8	116	6.1	9.9	0.6	ns	
Abscess/pyomyositis	14	87	10.7	7.4	1.4	ns	
Extremities other	6	48	4.6	4.1	1.1	ns	

* Incidence rate is calculated per 100 person years of follow-up. The number of person years of follow-up was 130.7 in men with and 1168.1 in men without HIV-1 infection. Relative risk is the ratio and attributable risk is the difference of the incidence rates in those with and without HIV-1 infection.

** ns is not significant (P>0.05)

The total number of diagnoses per year of follow-up in HIV-1 infected and non-HIV-1 infected men was 7.2 and 5.7 respectively (RR 1.3, P<0.0001); in women these numbers were 6.6 and 6.1 respectively (RR 1.1, P>0.05). The crude population etiological fraction was 2.5%.

A number of clinical diagnoses were significantly more common among men with than in men without HIV-1 infection (Table 3). Attributable risks (AR) of more than 10/100 person-years were found in men for the clinical diagnoses of fever (AR 32.4/100 pyr), bacterial skin infections (AR 11.4/100), tonsillitis/ sore throat (AR 16.1/100), diarrhoea (AR 17.8/100), and dysentery (AR 21.0/100). The highest relative risks were found for the association between HIV-1 infection and herpes zoster (RR 20.9), orchitis/epididimitis (RR 5.0), and bacterial skin infections (RR 2.8). The clinical diagnosis of hypertension was found to be less common among HIV-1 infected men (RR 0.0). However, at regular follow-up, there was no negative association between HIV-1

Table 4. The incidence of abnormal laboratory findings in a cohort of 1478 male factory workers

Laboratory findings	Number of cases		Incidence rate*		Relative risk	P-value**	Attributable rist (/100 pyr)
	HIV+	HIV-	HIV+	HIV-			
Blood smear							
Malaria parasites	34	168	26.0	14.4	1.8	<0.01	11.6
Number examined	123	853	94.1	73.0	1.3	<0.01	21.1
Stool smear							
Hookworm	25	269	19.1	23.0	0.8	ns	
T saginata	0	6	0.0	0.5	0.0	ns	
A lumbricoides	2	20	1.5	1.7	0.9	ns	
G lamblia	11	41	8.4	3.5	2.4	<0.05	4.9
E histolytica	28	157	21.4	13.4	1.6	<0.05	8.0
S mansoni	12	82	9.2	7.0	1.3	ns	
S stercoralis	11	66	8.4	5.7	1.5	ns	
T hominis	12	49	9.2	4.2	2.2	<0.05	5.0
White blood cells	12	60	9.2	5.1	1.8	ns	
Number examined	251	1794	192.1	153.6	1.3	0.001	38.5
Urine chemistry							
Albumen	4	42	3.1	3.6	0.9	ns	
Number examined	9	55	6.9	4.7	1.5	ns	
Urine sediment							
S haematobium	4	46	3.1	3.9	0.8	ns	
White blood cells	51	310	39.0	26.5	1.5	<0.05	12.5
Red blood cells	20	111	15.3	9.5	1.6	ns	
Number examined	80	505	61.2	43.2	1.4	<0.01	18.0
Smear genital discharge							
Gram-negative diplococci seen intracellularly	5	9	3.8	0.8	5.0	<0.01	3.0
Number examined	7	30	5.4	2.6	2.1	ns	

* Incidence rate is calculated per 100 person years of follow-up of the total study population. The number of person years of follow-up was 130.7 in men with and 1168.1 in men without HIV-1 infection. Relative risk is the ratio and attributable risk is the difference of the incidence rates in those with and without HIV-1 infection.

** ns is not significant (P>0.05)

infection and the prevalence or incidence of a blood pressure of 160 mm Hg or more systolic or 100 mm Hg or more diastolic.

HIV-1 infection was associated with a low body mass index (BMI). At first measurement a BMI of less than 18 kg/m^2 was found in 20/129 (15.5%) of men with and 80/1,114 (7.2%) of those without HIV-1 infection (OR 2.2; 95% CI 1.3–3.6). At

Table 5. Malaria parasitaemia in 976 blood slides from febrile patients in a cohort of 1446 male factory workers who never received a blood transfusion

Number of parasites (in total fields containing 200 WBC)	Number (%)		OR (95% CI)
	HIV+	HIV-	
0	88 (73.9)	667 (80.4)	1
1-3	3 (2.5)	36 (4.3)	0.6 (0.2-2.1)
4-15	18 (15.1)	101 (12.2)	1.4 (0.8-2.3)
16+	10 (8.4)	26 (3.1)	2.9 (1.4-6.3)
Total	123 (100.0)	853 (100.0)	

χ^2 9.7, 3 df; P=0.02 χ^2 trend 5.7; P=0.02

follow-up the incidence rates for developing a BMI of less than 18 kg/m^2 was 7.7 and 2.6 per 100 pyr respectively (RR 3.0; Z=2.33, P<0.05).

At first measurement HIV-1 infection was strongly associated with anaemia (haemoglobin <10 gr/dl) in men (OR 2.6; 95% CI 1.6–4.3). At follow-up anaemia was more likely to develop in HIV-1 infected men (RR 3.4, Z=3.64, P<0.001). The following laboratory findings were also significantly more common among men infected with HIV-1 than in those not infected with HIV-1 (Table 4): *Malaria parasitaemia* (RR 1.8), *E histolytica* (RR 1.6), *G intestinalis* (RR 2.4) and *T hominis* (RR 2.2) infections, white blood cells in the urine (RR 1.5), and intracellular gram-negative diplococci in a smear of genital discharge (RR 5.0). Laboratory examinations of stools, urine sediment, and blood smear for detection of malaria parasitaemia were performed significantly more frequently in men with than in men without HIV-1 infection. Among the blood slides examined higher levels of malaria parasitaemia were found in those of HIV-1 infected men than in those without HIV-1 infection (Table 5). A similar trend was found in women, but this was not statistically significant. Those ever having received a blood transfusion were excluded from Table 5, although this exclusion made little difference to the results.

In women numbers were much smaller with 38.6 person-years of follow-up in those with and 194.5 person-years in those without HIV-1 infection. The only clinical diagnoses significantly associated with HIV-1 infection were herpes zoster (RR 10.1, AR 9.4), diarrhoea (RR 1.9, AR 23.0), and genital discharge (RR 2.3, AR 14.6). The only laboratory result significantly associated with HIV-1 infection in women was S stercoralis infection (RR 12.6, AR 12.0).

Discussion

This study has shown that 62% of mortality was attributable to HIV-1, implying that HIV-1 was the major cause of death in this adult population with an HIV-1 prevalence of 12% and an annual HIV-1 incidence of 1.2%. HIV-1 contributed to an substantially increased morbidity for a relatively small number of clinical diagnoses; overall, only

2.5% of clinical diagnoses were attributable to HIV-1.

The incidence rate of HIV-1 infection in this study was similar to that in an occupational cohort in Zaire [20,21], and rural population cohorts in Uganda [12,22], but much lower than that in an urban population in a neighbouring Region in Tanzania [23], urban women of childbearing age in Rwanda and Zambia [24,25], or high risk groups in Africa such as spouses of HIV-1 infected people [26,27], prostitutes [28–30], and attenders of sexually transmitted disease clinics [31].

Information obtained from monitoring HIV-1 prevalence in pregnant women has suggested that this prevalence has been stable since 1989 in Mwanza town [32]. The present study is consistent with the hypothesis that the HIV-1 epidemic has reached a steady state in this urban population, as the number of HIV-1 seroconversions was only slightly larger than that of HIV-1 associated deaths.

Mortality rates in those with and without HIV-1 infection were similar to those reported from Rwanda [11] and Uganda [12]. The population etiological fraction in the present study (62%) was lower than that in Rwanda (90%), which is explained by the difference in HIV-1 prevalence (12% and 33% respectively). However, it is striking that at an HIV-1 prevalence of 12%, 62% of deaths in adults were attributable to HIV-1 infection, making it the most important public health problem in this adult population. It seems likely that a sizable proportion of deaths (at least 21%) occurred in HIV-1 infected people who had not yet developed AIDS, as was shown among intravenous drug users in the U.S. [33–35], although because of data limitations a precise estimate of this proportion could not be made. Tuberculosis was diagnosed in 2 out of 14 deaths; an autopsy study in Ivory Coast [36] suggests that a much larger proportion of deaths in the study population may be attributable to tuberculosis than is evident from our data.

As in Uganda, only a small fraction of overall morbidity was attributable to HIV-1, perhaps partly because of a high level of background morbidity [37]. However, the present study suggests that HIV-1 is contributing substantially to the incidence of fever, bacterial skin infections, tonsillitis/sore throat, diarrhoea, dysentery, urethral discharge, low body mass index, and anaemia. Laboratory investigations suggest that some of the infections contributing to this increased incidence may be malaria (mainly *P falciparum* in this area) in the case of fever, *E histolytica, G intestinalis, T hominis*, and *S stercoralis* in the case of diarrhoea and dysentery, and N gonorrhoea in the case of urethral discharge.

The study has a number of limitations. Although total enrolment was reasonable at 87% of those eligible, losses to follow-up were considerable at 27% after two years. These losses to follow-up were largely due to two factors: many study participants did not like to repeatedly submit blood samples, and due to economic difficulties the factory had to temporarily close down in the second year of the study, sending staff on unpaid leave. The first factor might be partly overcome by more intensive follow-up and education; the latter factor however, which affected in particular those in younger age groups, is much more serious, and may if repeated jeopardize the continuation of this cohort study.

The data on morbidity have various limitations. The most important are probably self-selection of patients and classification errors in the conditions listed. Selection bias is likely to be largest for conditions people prefer to have treated in hospital, by traditional healers, or self-treatment, and is likely to be different for different diseases. This bias would be smallest for results from routine measurements such as anaemia and body mass index. The size of the selection bias might for selected conditions be estimated by enquiring about disease episodes inbetween regular follow-up visits.

Misclassification of diseases is likely to be mainly due to differences in diagnoses made by different assistant medical officers and limited diagnostic facilities in the study clinic. As the assistant medical officers did not know whether or not patients had HIV-1 infection, knowledge of HIV-1 status is unlikely to be a major source of bias. Random misclassification would tend to reduce differences in disease incidence between those with and without HIV-1 infection, and therefore would not invalidate the associations found. Classification errors can for selected conditions be reduced by specific training of staff and the use of standardized interview, examination, and laboratory procedures. These data present a basis for selecting the conditions into which such further research in this cohort seems to be useful.

Another limitation of the results on HIV-1 associated morbidity is that they are based on a large number of comparisons, which would lead to some significant associations just by chance: of the 44 comparisons in Table 3 and the 20 comparisons in Table 4, 2 and 1 respectively would be expected to be significant (P<0.05) by chance. However, it is obvious that this does not explain all the associations found.

Associations have been described previously between HIV-1 infection and diarrhoeal diseases, loss of weight, herpes zoster, bacterial skin infections, anaemia, and fever [15,38–44]. Oral thrush has been shown to be associated with HIV-1 [38,39,45] and may partially explain the increased incidence of tonsillitis/sore throat. There is conflicting evidence on whether the incidence of genital discharge is increased in those with HIV-1 infection [46]; this study suggests that the incidence *is* increased. The negative association between HIV-1 infection and clinically diagnosed hypertension in men was not confirmed by routine measurements of blood pressure in the total study population, and is unlikely to be of great importance.

In diarrhoeal diseases a limited number of treatable pathogens were associated with HIV-1 infection. This suggests some HIV-1 associated diarrhoea may be amenable to treatment of the causative organism. However, in the majority of cases no such organism was identified, also not in a period when cultures were done for bacterial pathogens (data not shown), which is in line with experience elsewhere [15,47].

Incidences based on field laboratory results may be biased as most tests were performed on request. For instance, because patients with HIV-1 infection have more frequent episodes of fever, they are more frequently examined for the presence of malaria parasitaemia. However, there are two arguments supporting the association between HIV-1 and malaria. If there were no association between HIV-1 infection and malaria, the proportion of positive thick films might be expected to be *lower* in those with HIV-1 infection because of the higher incidence of fever in this group attributable to other causes: the opposite was found. In addition, the level of parasitaemia in the slides examined was higher in those with HIV-1 infection.

A limitation of counting parasites against white blood cells is that the total white cell count tends to drop with progressing immunodeficiency, in particular because of dropping CD4 lymphocyte counts. However, this is unlikely to fully explain the differences in parasite levels between those with and without HIV-1 infection in the present study, as the adjacent categories in Table 5 represent a fourfold difference in parasite counts.

The association between HIV-1 infection and P falciparum malaria would potentially be of major importance as both infections are widespread, in particular in Africa. Theoretically it might be expected that HIV-1 infection in its advanced stages would lead to higher levels of malaria parasitaemia or more serious malarial disease, because of the role of CD4 lymphocytes in immunity against malaria and the decline of CD4 in the course of HIV-1 infection [48,49]. Antibody levels against synthetic P falciparum ring stage peptide were shown to be lower in AIDS patients than in controls [50].

However, in cross-sectional studies no association was found between asymptomatic malaria parasitaemia and HIV-1 infection [51], nor between clinical malaria and HIV-1 infection in hospital patients [52–55] or in those deceased in hospital [36,56]. Prospective studies showed a few positive findings including an increased incidence of fever with malaria parasitaemia in HIV-1 infected people (which might be partly explained by ascertainment bias) [57], a non-significant relative risk for getting malaria of 1.6 in young children with AIDS [58], and an increased geometric mean parasite density in children with HIV-1 infection [59].

An association between HIV-1 infection and malaria appears to be present but appears not to be very strong. In addition to the variables included in the present study, future studies should include measurement of self-treatment with antimalarials and of the degree of immunodeficiency. Total white blood counts would need to be measured as well to obtain parasite counts per volume unit of blood.

Acknowledgements

We thank the Principal Secretary, Ministry of Health and the Director General, National Institute for Medical Research for permission to carry out the study and to publish its results. We are grateful to Prof A S Muller, Prof R A Coutinho, and Dr J T Boerma for their critical comments on drafts of this paper.
The research for this publication was financed by the Netherlands' Minister for Development Cooperation, Section for Research and Technology, P.O.Box 20061, 2500 EB, The Hague, as part of the Tanzania-Netherlands Research Project on AIDS and HIV Infection in Mwanza Region. Responsibility for the contents and for the opinions expressed rests solely with the authors; publication does not constitute an endorsement by the Netherlands' Minister for Development Co-operation.

References

1. Dixon DO, Rida WN, Fast PE, Hoth DF. HIV vaccine trials: some design issues including sample size calculation. J Acquir Immune Defic Syndr 1993;6:485-496.

2. Nkowane BJ. Prevalence and incidence of HIV infection in Africa: a review of data published in 1990. AIDS 1991;5(Suppl 1):S7-S15.

3. Ryder RW, Piot P. Epidemiology of HIV-1 infection in Africa. Bailliere's Clinical Tropical Medicine and Communicable Diseases 1988;3:13-29.

4. De Cock KM et al. AIDS - the leading cause of death in the west African city of Abidjan, Ivory Coast. Science 1990;249:793-796.

5. De Cock KM, Porter A, Odehouri K, et al. Rapid emergence of AIDS in Abidjan, Ivory Coast. Lancet 1989;ii:408-411.

6. Gilks CF, Brindle RJ, Otieno LS, et al. Life-threatening bacteraemia in HIV-1 seropositive adults admitted to hospital in Nairobi, Kenya. Lancet 1990;336:545-549.

7. Hassig SE Perriens J, Baende E, et al. An analysis of the economic impact of HIV infection among patients at Mama Yemo Hospital, Kinshasa, Zaire. AIDS 1990;4:883-887.

8. Mbaga JM, Pallangyo KJ, Bakari M, Aris EA. Survival time of patients with acquired immune deficiency syndrome: experience with 274 patients in Dar-es-Salaam. East Afr Med J 1990;67:95-99.

9. Nelson AM et al, Hassig SE, Kayembe M, et al. HIV-1 seropositivity and mortality at University Hospital, Kinshasa, Zaire,1987. AIDS 1991;5:583-586.

10. Muller O, Moser R. HIV-1 disease in a Kampala hospital 1985-89 (letter) Lancet 1990;335:236-237.

11. Lindan CP, Allen S, Serufilira A, et al. Predictors of mortality among HIV-infected women in Kigali, Rwanda. Ann Intern Med 1992;116:320-328.

12. Mulder DW, Nunn AJ, Wagner HU, Kamali A, Kengeya-Kayondo JF. HIV-1 incidence and HIV-1-associated mortality in a rural Ugandan population cohort. AIDS 1994;8:87-92.

13. Anderson RM, May RM, Boily MC, Garnett GP, Rowley JT. The spread of HIV-1 in Africa: sexual contact patterns and the predicted demographic impact of AIDS. Nature 1991;352:581-589.

14. Anderson RM. Some aspects of sexual behaviour and the potential demographic impact of AIDS in developing countries. Soc Sci Med 1992;34:271-280.)

15. Colebunders RL, Latif AS. Natural history and clinical presentation of HIV-1 infection in adults. AIDS 1991;5(Suppl 1):S103-S112.

16. Barongo LR, Borgdorff MW, Mosha FF, et al. The epidemiology of HIV-1 infection in urban areas, roadside settlements and rural villages in Mwanza Region, Tanzania. AIDS 1992;6:1521-1528.

17. Barongo LR, Borgdorff MW, Newell JN, et al. Intake of a cohort study of urban factory workers in northwest Tanzania: risk factors for HIV-1 infection. Trop Geograph Med 1994; 46:157-162.

18. World Health Organization. Acquired Immune Deficiency Syndrome (AIDS) - Proposed WHO criteria for interpreting results from Western blot assays for HIV-1, HIV-2, and HTLV-I/HTLV-II. Wkly Epidemiol Rec 1990;65:281-283.

19. World Health Organization. Acquired immunodeficiency syndrome (AIDS) - WHO/CDC case definition for AIDS. Wkly Epidemiol Rec 1986;61:69-73.

20. Mann JM, Francis H, Quinn TC, et al. HIV seroincidence in a hospital worker population. Ann Soc Belg Med Trop 1986;66:245-250.

21. N'galy B, Ryder RW, Bila K, et al. Human immunodeficiency virus infection among employees in an African hospital. New Engl J Med 1988;319:1123-1127.

22. Wawer MJ, Sewankambo NK, Berkley S, et al. Incidence of HIV-1 infection in a rural region of Uganda. BMJ 1994;308:171-173.

23. Killewo JZJ, Sandstrom A, Bredberg Raden U, Mhalu FS, Biberfeld G, Wall S. Incidence of HIV-1 infection among adults in the Kagera Region of Tanzania. Int J Epidemiol 1993;22:528-536.

24. Hira SK, Mangrola SG, Mwale C, et al. Apparent vertical transmission of human immunodeficiency

virus type 1 by breastfeeding in Zambia. J Pediatr 1990;117:421-424.

25. Allen S, Serufilira A, Bogaerts J, et al. Confidential HIV testing and condom promotion in Africa. JAMA 1992;268:3338-3343.

26. Allen S, Tice J, Perre P van de, et al. Effect of serotesting with counselling on condom use and seroconversion among HIV discordant couples in Africa. BMJ 1992;304:1605-1609.

27. Kamenga M, Ryder RW, Jingu M, et al. Evidence of marked sexual behaviour change associated with low HIV-1 seroconversion in 149 married couples with discordant HIV-1 serostatus: experience at an HIV counselling center in Zaire. AIDS 1991;5:61-67.

28. Plummer FA, Simonsen JN, Cameron DW, et al. Cofactors in male-female sexual transmission of human immunodeficiency virus type 1. J Infect Dis 1991;163:233-239.

29. Laga M, Manoka A, Kivuvu M, et al. Non-ulcerative sexually transmitted diseases as risk factors for HIV-1 transmission in women: results from a cohort study. AIDS 1993;7:95-102.

30. Zekeng L, Feldblum PJ, Oliver RM, Kaptue L. Barrier contraceptive use and HIV, infection among high-risk women in Cameroon. AIDS 1993;7:725-731.

31. Cameron DW, Simonsen JN, D'Costa LJ, et al. Female to male transmission of human immunodeficiency virus type 1: risk factors for seroconversion in men. Lancet 1989;ii:403-407.

32. Kigadye RM, Klokke A, Nicoll A, et al. Sentinel surveillance for HIV-1 among pregnant women in a developing country: 3 years experience and comparison with a population survey. AIDS 1993;7:849-855.

33. Stoneburner RL, Des Jarlais DC, Benezra D, et al. A larger spectrum of severe HIV-1-related disease in intravenous drug users in New York City. Science 1988;242:916-919.

34. Selwyn PA. Injection drug use, mortality, and the AIDS epidemic. Am J Public Health 1991;81:1247-1249.

35. Selwyn PA, Alcabes P, Hartel D, et al. Clinical manifestations and predictors of disease progression in drug users with human immunodeficiency virus infection. N Engl J Med 1992;327:1697-1703.

36. Lucas SB, Hounnou A, Peacock C, et al. The mortality and pathology of HIV infection in a West African city. AIDS 1993;7:1569-1579.

37. Wagner HU, Kamali A, Nunn AJ, Kengeya-Kayondo JF, Mulder DW. General and HIV-1-associated morbidity in a rural Ugandan community. AIDS 1993;7:1461-1467.

38. Melbye M, Njelesani EK, Bayley A, et al. Evidence for heterosexual transmission and clinical manifestations of human immunodeficiency virus infection and related conditions in Lusaka, Zambia. Lancet 1986;ii:1113-1115.

39. Colebunders RL, Mann JM, Francis H, et al. Evaluation of a clinical case-definition of acquired immunodeficiency syndrome in Africa. Lancet 1987;i:492-494.

40. Conlon CP, Pinching AJ, Perera CU, Moody A, Luo NP, Lucas SB. HIV-related enteropathy in Zambia: a clinical, microbiological and histological study. Am J Trop Med Hyg 1990;42:83-88.

41. Colebunders R, Francis H, Mann JM, et al. Persistent diarrhea strongly associated with HIV infection in Kinshasa, Zaire. Am J Gastroenterol 1987;82:859-864.

42. Colebunders R, Mann JM, Francis H, et al. Herpes zoster in African patients: a clinical predictor of human immunodeficiency virus infection. J Infect Dis 1988;157:314-318.

43. Perre P van de, Bakkers E, Batungwanayo J, et al. Herpes zoster in African patients: an early manifestation of HIV infection. Scand J Infect Dis 1988;20:277-282.

44. Dehne KL, Dhlakama DG, Richter C, Mawadza M, McClean D, Huss R. Herpes zoster as an indicator of HIV infection in Africa. Trop Doctor 1992;22:68-70.

45. Magaruka Z, Perriens JH, Kapita B, Piot P. Oral manifestations of HIV-1 infection in Zairian patients

(letter). AIDS 1991;5:237-238.

46. Laga M, Nzila N, Goeman J. The interrelationship of sexually transmitted diseases and HIV infection: implications for the control of both epidemics in Africa. AIDS 1991;5(Suppl 1):S55-S63.

47. Colebunders R, Lusakumuni K, Nelson AM, et al. Persistent diarrhoea in Zairian AIDS patients: an endoscopic and histological study. Gut 1988;29:1687-1691.

48. Butcher GA. HIV and malaria: a lesson in immunology? Parasitology Today 1992;8:307-311.

49. Lucas SB. Missing infections in AIDS. Trans Roy Soc Trop Med Hyg 1990;84(Suppl 1):34-38.

50. Wabwire-Mangen F, Shiff CJ, Vlahov D, et al. Immunological effects of HIV-1 infection on the humoral response to malaria in an African population. Am J Trop Med Hyg 1989;45:504-511.

51. Allen S, Van de perre P, Serufilira A, et al. Human immunodeficiency virus and malaria in a representative sample of childbearing women in Kigali, Rwanda. J Infect Dis 1991;164:67-71.

52. Muller O, Musoke P, Sen G, Moser R. Pediatric HIV-1 disease in a Kampala hospital. J Trop Pediatr 1990;36:283-286.

53. Muller O, Moser R. The clinical and parasitological presentation of Plasmodium falciparum malaria is unaffected by HIV-1 infection. Trans Roy Soc trop Med Hyg 1990;84:336-338.

54. Simooya OO, Mwendapole RM, Siziya S, Fleming AF. Relation between falciparum malaria and HIV seropositivity in Ndola, Zambia. Br Med J 1988;297:30-31.

55. Simooya OO, Mwendapole RM, Sikateyo BM. Severe falciparum malaria and the acquired immunodeficiency syndrome (AIDS) in Zambia (letter). Ann Trop Med Parasitol 1991;85:269-270.

56. Muller O, Moser R, Guggenberger P, Alexander M. AIDS in Africa (letter). New Engl J Med 1991;324:847-848

57. Colebunders R, Bahwe Y, Nekwei W, et al. Incidence of malaria and efficacy of oral quinine in patients recently infected with human immunodeficiency virus in Kinshasa, Zaire. J Infection 1990;21:167-173.

58. Greenberg AE, Nsa W, Ryder RW, et al. Plasmodium falciparum malaria and perinatally acquired human immunodeficiency virus type 1 infection in Kinshasa, Zaire. New Engl J Med 1991;325:105-109.

59. Shaffer N, Hedberg K, Davachi F, et al. Trends and risk factors for HIV-1 seropositivity among outpatient children, Kinshasa, Zaire. AIDS 1990;4:1231-1236.

60. Nguyen-Dinh P, Greenberg AE, Mann JM, et al. Absence of association between Plasmodium falciparum malaria and human immunodeficiency virus infection in children in Kinshasa, Zaire. Bull World Hlth Org 1987;65:607-613.

61. Greenberg AE, Nguyen-Dinh P, Mann JM, et al. The association between malaria, blood transfusions, and HIV seropositivity in a pediatric population in Kinshasa, Zaire. JAMA 1988;259:545-549.

62. Morrow RH, Colebunders RL, Chin J. Interactions of HIV infection with endemic tropical diseases. AIDS 1989;3(Suppl 1):S79-S87.

10

General discussion

The study presented in this thesis was planned as follows: first the prevalence of and risk factors for HIV-1 infection (and other STDs) would be determined in a representative population sample, which was stratified by urban, roadside, and rural residence. Information on HIV-1 prevalence from this survey would be used amongst other purposes to validate information on HIV-1 prevalence from routine surveillance by the Tanzania National AIDS Control Programme.

Thereafter, a cohort study would be set up in Mwanza Municipality in order to (1) determine the incidence of HIV-1 infection and other STDs, (2) identify risk factors for HIV-1 seroconversion and for contracting other STDs, (3) document changes in risk behaviour, in particular condom use and partner change, after the introduction of interventions, (4) determine whether changes in reported risk behaviour are associated with a reduced incidence of HIV-1 and other STDs and (5) describe the natural history of HIV-1 infection.

The population survey (Chapter 3) provided baseline information before embarking on two large HIV-1 intervention research programmes: TANERA and AMREF's (African Medical and Research Foundation) STD/HIV intervention trial. The latter aimed to demonstrate the impact of a regionwide STD control programme on HIV-1 transmission, while the former aimed to develop and evaluate interventions for the reduction of sexual partner change, promotion of condom use, and reduction of medical care related transmission. The survey results were used in the further planning of both projects. An example of the usefulness of the survey data for the cohort study is given in Chapter 7: before the factory cohort study was started, it was suggested that factory workers might be an unrepresentative group, being at much lower risk than the general urban population. A comparison with the population survey results suggests that this is not the case. In addition, the study represents one of the few published representative population surveys of HIV-1 infection in Africa [1–4)] or, indeed, in the world.

Sentinel surveillance of HIV-1 prevalence in selected population groups such as blood donors and pregnant women is recommended by the World Health Organization and used by the Tanzania National AIDS Control Programme as a method to monitor the HIV-1 epidemic. A problem with sentinel surveillance is that the representativeness of the sentinel groups is often unknown. Therefore, extrapolation of results from sentinel groups to the general population may not be justified.

The validation of sentinel surveillance (Chapter 4) was reassuring in that data from blood donors appeared to be fairly representative. This is important because the National AIDS Control Programme uses HIV-1 prevalence among blood donors to estimate prevalence in the total population. It is also relevant to investigators who use blood donors as controls in case-control studies which aim to show that HIV-1 infection is a risk factor for the development of the disease being studied. Data from antenatal clinic attenders, however, produced an underestimate of population HIV-1 prevalence.

In this study, the representativeness of various sentinel groups was determined at one point in time. It is also important to assess the validity of using various sentinel groups for monitoring *trends*. This would require a repeated comparison between HIV-1 prevalence in sentinel groups and a representative population sample, which might be carried out for instance five years after the first comparison presented in Chapter 4.

Data from the population survey were also combined with data from the tuberculosis/ leprosy programme in order to determine the risk of HIV-1 infection for developing active tuberculosis or leprosy. The study on the association of HIV-1 and tuberculosis disease showed that the relative risk of HIV-1 infection for the development of active tuberculosis was 8.3 and that 29% of tuberculosis cases in Mwanza Region were attributable to HIV-1 infection. The large increase in the number of tuberculosis cases in Mwanza Region over the past 10 years is most likely attributable to HIV-1 infection (Chapter 5). It seems likely that with the increase in the incidence of sputum smear-positive tuberculosis also the annual risk of tuberculosis infection will increase. Therefore, eventually people without HIV-1 infection may become increasingly at risk for developing tuberculosis disease.

A novel finding was the association of HIV-1 infection and multibacillary leprosy (Chapter 6). This association was expected to be present on theoretical grounds because a reduced cellular immunity, which occurs with the progress of HIV-1 infection, is associated with multibacillary leprosy and because there is an association between HIV-1 infection and other diseases due to mycobacteria, in particular *M. tuberculosis*. Though the association had previously been shown only in one small hospital based study [5], it had not been confirmed by larger studies elsewhere [6,7,8] and the results of the first study have been questioned due to hospital bias [6]. Chapter 6 presents the first community-based study demonstrating this association.

The public health implications of the association between HIV-1 infection and multibacillary leprosy are thus far limited, because leprosy occurs mainly in rural areas and HIV-1 infection in urban areas. With the increasing spread of HIV-1 infection in rural areas, the public health importance of the association is likely to increase. If relapses of leprosy are also more common in HIV-1 infected people, as suggested by Pönnighaus *et al.* [6], this might further increase the problem of leprosy control. In the past 10 years the prevalence of leprosy has been reduced drastically because of the use of multi-drug therapy. Hopefully, the interaction with HIV-1 infection will not prove a stumbling block in the further control of this disease.

At intake for the cohort study, which was carried out among factory workers and their spouses, HIV-1 prevalence and risk factors for HIV-1 infection were found to be similar to those in the general population, and cooperation of the factory workers was found to be good (Chapter 7). At intake it was also shown that sexual partner change occurs frequently, condoms are seldom used, and a large proportion of sexual partner change takes place outside the setting of commercial sex workers, which has implications for focusing interventions (Chapter 8).

After two years of follow-up, the incidence of HIV-1 in the cohort was found to be 1.2 per 100 person-years (Chapter 9), which is similar to that in an occupational cohort in Zaire [9,10] and rural population cohorts in Uganda [11,12], but much lower than that in an urban population in a neighbouring region in Tanzania [13], urban women of childbearing age in Rwanda and Zambia [14,15], or high-risk groups in Africa such as spouses of HIV-1-infected people [16,17], prostitutes [18–20], and attenders of STD clinics [21]. The estimated incidence at intake of 1.4% was close to measured incidence at follow-up of 1.2%, suggesting that the method of estimation used at intake was appropriate. Presently, the number of seroconversions is too small to relate them to risk factors. As HIV-1 infection has a low incidence and the sexual risk behaviour in a population changes only slowly, the cohort study needs to continue for a longer time and be expanded in size to increase statistical power.

HIV-1-associated mortality in the cohort was shown to be great: 62% of deaths in this adult population were attributable to HIV-1 infection, making HIV-1 by far the most important cause of death. High levels of mortality attributable to HIV-1 infection have now been well documented in Africa in prospective studies in Rwanda [22], Uganda [11], and Tanzania (Chapter 9). Recent scepticism on whether HIV is a major cause of death in Africa* is not supported by research results.

The cohort study also showed that among patients with fever, HIV-1-infected individuals had a higher proportion of blood slides positive for malaria parasites, and higher levels of parasitaemia (Chapter 9). The interaction of malaria and HIV-1 is potentially important as both infections are widespread, particularly in Africa. Theoretically, it might be expected that HIV-1 infection in its advanced stages would lead to higher levels of malaria parasitaemia and/or more serious malarial disease, because of the role of CD4 lymphocytes in immunity against malaria and the decline of CD4 in the course of HIV-1 infection [23].

In cross-sectional studies no association was found between asymptomatic malaria parasitaemia and HIV-1 infection [24], nor between clinical malaria and HIV-1 infection in hospital patients [25–28])or in those who died in hospital [29,30]. On the other hand, prospective studies showed an increased incidence of fever with malaria parasitaemia

---

* See for instance:
  - Steve Connor. HIV is Africa's big killer. Independent on Sunday, 14-11-93.
  - The African AIDS 'lie'. Item 727. AIDS Newsletter 1993;8(12):7.
  - Anver Versi, Baffour Ankomah. AIDS: the epidemic that never was. New African, December 1993:8-11.
  - Impact. Vara televisie 2-12-93.
  - Gerbrand Feenstra. De lezers van de Sunday Times krijgen geen aids. Volkskrant 4-12-93.
  - Aids-Coordinatiegroep. TV informeert onjuist over aids. Parool 7-12-93.
  - Joke Mat. 'Mythe' aids in Afrika roeit generatie uit. NRC Handelsblad 31-12-93.
  - Aids-epidemie in Afrika ontkend. Onze Wereld, januari 1994.

in HIV-1 infected people [31], a non-significant relative risk for getting malaria of 1.6 in young children with AIDS [32], and an increased geometric mean parasite density in children with HIV-1 infection [33].

These studies, including the one presented in Chapter 9, seem to suggest that an association between HIV-1 infection and malaria exists but that it is not very strong. In addition to the variables included in the cohort study so far, future studies should include measurement of self-treatment with antimalarials and of immunodeficiency (by doing CD4 counts). The cohort study would also benefit greatly from a capacity to do CD4 counts for studies on (predictors of) mortality and on the risk of HIV-1 infection for developing diseases other than malaria.

In conclusion, the studies completed so far have determined the prevalence of and risk factors for HIV-1 infection in a representative population sample in Mwanza Region; evaluated the HIV-1 sentinel surveillance system; determined the relative risk associated with HIV-1 infection for the development of tuberculosis and leprosy disease; described HIV-1 prevalence and risk factors as well as sexual partner change and condom use in a predominantly male factory population; and determined HIV-1 incidence and HIV-1 associated mortality and morbidity in a predominantly male factory population.

A major challenge for the project in the near future is to measure the effectiveness and impact of interventions aiming at reducing sexual transmission of HIV-1 infection (and other sexually transmitted diseases) through a reduction of sexual partner change and condom promotion. In addition, it should provide further crucial information on the natural history of HIV-1 infection in Africa in men *and* women.

References

1. Rwandan HIV Seroprevalence Study Group. Nationwide community-based serologicalsurvey of HIV-1 and other human retrovirus infections in a Central African country. Lancet 1989;i:941-943.
2. Killewo J, Nyamuryekunge K, Sandström A, et al. Prevalence of HIV-1 infection in the Kagera region of Tanzania: a population-based study. AIDS 1990;4:1081-1085.
3. Wawer MJ, Serwadda D, Musgrave SD, Konde-Lulu JK, Musagara M, Sewankambo NK. Dynamics of spread of HIV-1 infection in a rural district of Uganda. BMJ 1991;303:1303-1306.
4. Nunn AJ, Kengeya-Kayondo JF, Malamba SS, Seeley JA, Mulder DW. Risk factors for HIV-1 infection in adults in a rural Ugandan community: a population study. AIDS 1994;8:81-86.
5. Meeran K. Prevalence of HIV infection among patients with leprosy and tuberculosis in rural Zambia. BMJ 1989;298:364-365.
6. Pönnighaus JM, Mwanjasi LJ, Fine PEM, et al. Is HIV infection a risk factor for leprosy? Int J Lepr 1991;59:221-228.
7. Leonard G, Sangare A, Verdier M, et al. Prevalence of HIV infection among patients with leprosy in African countries and Yemen. J Acq Imm Def Syndr 1990;3:1109-1113.
8. Tekle-Haimanot R, Frommel D, Tadesse T, Verdier M, Abebe M, Denis F. A survey of HTLV-1 and HIVs in Ethiopian leprosy patients. AIDS 1991;5:108-110.
9. Mann JM, Francis H, Quinn TC, et al. HIV seroincidence in a hospital worker population. Ann Soc Belg Med Trop 1986;66:245-250.

10. N'galy B, Ryder RW, Bila K, et al. Human immunodeficiency virus infection among employees in an African hospital. New Engl J Med 1988;319:1123-1127.
11. Mulder DW, Nunn AJ, Wagner HU, Kamali A, Kengeya-Kayondo JF. HIV-1 incidence and HIV-1-associated mortality in a rural Ugandan population cohort. AIDS 1994;8:87-92.
12. Wawer MJ, Sewankambo NK, Berkley S, et al. Incidence of HIV-1 infection in a rural region of Uganda. BMJ 1994;308:171-173.
13. Killewo JZJ, Sandstrom A, Bredberg Raden U, Mhalu FS, Biberfeld G, Wall S. Incidence of HIV-1 infection among adults in the Kagera Region of Tanzania. Int J Epidemiol 1993;22:528-536.
14. Hira SK, Mangrola SG, Mwale C, et al. Apparent vertical transmission of human immunodeficiency virus type 1 by breastfeeding in Zambia. J Pediatr 1990;117:421-424.
15. Allen S, Serufilira A, Bogaerts J, et al. Confidential HIV testing and condom promotion in Africa. JAMA 1992;268:3338-3343.
16. Allen S, Tice J, Perre P van de, et al. Effect of serotesting with counselling on condom use and seroconversion among HIV discordant couples in Africa. BMJ 1992;304:1605-1609.
17. Kamenga M, Ryder RW, Jingu M, et al. Evidence of marked sexual behaviour change associated with low HIV-1 seroconversion in 149 married couples with discordant HIV-1 serostatus: experience at an HIV counselling center in Zaire. AIDS 1991;5:61-67.
18. Plummer FA, Simonsen JN, Cameron DW, et al. Cofactors in male-female sexual transmission of human immunodeficiency virus type 1. J Infect Dis 1991;163:233-239.
19. Laga M, Manoka A, Kivuvu M, et al. Non-ulcerative sexually transmitted diseases as risk factors for HIV-1 transmission in women: results from a cohort study. AIDS 1993;7:95-102.
20. Zekeng L, Feldblum PJ, Oliver RM, Kaptue L. Barrier contraceptive use and HIV infection among high-risk women in Cameroon. AIDS 1993;7:725-731.
21. Cameron DW, Simonsen JN, D'Costa LJ, et al. Female to male transmission of human immunodeficiency virus type 1: risk factors for seroconversion in men. Lancet 1989;ii:403-407.
22. Lindan CP, Allen S, Serufilira A, et al. Predictors of mortality among HIV-infected women in Kigali, Rwanda. Ann Intern Med 1992;116:320-328.
23. Butcher GA. HIV and malaria: a lesson in immunology? Parasitology Today 1992;8:307-311.
24. Allen S, Van de perre P, Serufilira A, et al. Human immunodeficiency virus and malaria in a representative sample of childbearing women in Kigali, Rwanda. J Infect Dis 1991;164:67-71.
25. Muller O, Musoke P, Sen G, Moser R. Pediatric HIV-1 disease in a Kampala hospital. J Trop Pediatr 1990;36:283-286.
26. Muller O, Moser R. The clinical and parasitological presentation of Plasmodium falciparum malaria is unaffected by HIV-1 infection. Trans Roy Soc trop Med Hyg 1990;84:336-338.
27. Simooya OO, Mwendapole RM, Siziya S, Fleming AF. Relation between falciparum malaria and HIV seropositivity in Ndola, Zambia. Br Med J 1988;297:30-31.
28. Simooya OO, Mwendapole RM, Sikateyo BM. Severe falciparum malaria and the acquired immunodeficiency syndrome (AIDS) in Zambia (letter). Ann Trop Med Parasitol 1991;85:269-270.
29. Lucas SB, Hounnou A, Peacock C, et al. The mortality and pathology of HIV infection in a West African city. AIDS 1993;7:1569-1579.
30. Muller O, Moser R, Guggenberger P, Alexander M. AIDS in Africa (letter). New Engl J Med 1991;324:847-848
31. Colebunders R, Bahwe Y, Nekwei W, et al. Incidence of malaria and efficacy of oral quinine in patients recently infected with human immunodeficiency virus in Kinshasa, Zaire. J Infection 1990;21:167-173.

32. Greenberg AE, Nsa W, Ryder RW, et al. Plasmodium falciparum malaria and perinatally acquired human immunodeficiency virus type 1 infection in Kinshasa, Zaire. New Engl J Med 1991;325:105-109.
33. Shaffer N, Hedberg K, Davachi F, et al. Trends and risk factors for HIV-1 seropositivity among outpatient children, Kinshasa, Zaire. AIDS 1990;4:1231-1236.

Epidemiology of HIV-infection in Mwanza Region, Tanzania: summary

This thesis presents results from studies on the epidemiology of HIV-1 infection in adults in Mwanza Region, Tanzania. These studies were carried out as part of the Tanzania-Netherlands Research Project on HIV Infection in Mwanza Region, of which the author was the project leader.

In *Chapter 1* the literature is reviewed on the epidemiology of HIV-1 infection in adults in Africa. Within Africa there is much variation in the incidence of AIDS and in the prevalence and incidence of HIV-1 infection, thus far the problem is much greater in East than in West Africa. Limitations of information on HIV/AIDS prevalence and incidence include incomplete AIDS notification, selection bias in sentinel surveillance, and incomplete coverage of population surveys. Risk factors for heterosexual HIV-1 transmission are reviewed. They include sexual partner change, lack of condom use, other sexually transmitted diseases, a high viral load in the HIV-1 infected partner, sexual techniques, male circumcision, sex, age, urban/rural residence, mobility, and socioeconomic status. Interventions to reduce heterosexual HIV-1 transmission are presented: in particular, programmes to promote (1) behavioural change (reduction of sexual partner change), (2) condom use, and (3) early treatment of sexually transmitted diseases. Information on the natural history of HIV-1 infection in adults in Africa is reviewed, including aspects such as the incubation period, HIV-1-associated mortality, and HIV-1-associated morbidity, with special reference to the interaction of HIV-1 with tuberculosis, leprosy, and malaria.

Chapter 2 gives background information on Tanzania and Mwanza Region and describes the development, major activities, and organization of the Tanzania-Netherlands Research Project on HIV Infection in Mwanza Region. Tanzania is a low income country (GNP per capita $100) in East Africa. Mwanza Region is situated in the northwest of Tanzania along the shores of Lake Victoria and had a population in 1990 of 1,981,000. It functions as a trade centre in northwest Tanzania, as it is situated on trade routes to Uganda, Kenya, Rwanda, Burundi, and Dar es Salaam.

The first AIDS cases in Tanzania were notified in 1983. As a part of the response to the HIV/AIDS epidemic in Tanzania, the Tanzania-Netherlands Research Project on HIV infection in Mwanza Region started in 1990. The project aimed to contribute to the development of appropriate and effective methods for the reduction of HIV transmission through epidemiological, social-behavioural and clinical studies, and by carrying out pilot interventions. This thesis presents results of some of the epidemiological studies.

Chapter 3 describes a population survey in Mwanza Region carried out in 1990–1991 to determine the prevalence of HIV-1 infection among adults and to identify the most important risk factors. HIV-1 infection affected 2.5% of the adult population in rural villages, 7.3% in roadside settlements and 11.8% in town. It was 1.5 times more common in women than in men. HIV-1 occurred mostly in women aged 15–34 and in men aged 25–44. HIV-1 infection was associated with being separated or widowed, having multiple sexual partners, presence of syphilis antibodies, history of genital discharge or genital ulcer, travel to Mwanza town, and receiving injections during the past year. It was not associated with male circumcision. It was concluded that the results are consistent with spread of HIV-1 along the main roads.

In *Chapter 4* HIV-1 prevalence in various sentinel groups in the age group 15–54 years is compared with that of the general population in order to assess the validity of extrapolation from sentinel data. HIV-1 prevalence in the region, standardized by age, sex, and residence, was 4.1% (3.1% in non-urban areas and 11.4% in town). The standardized HIV-1 prevalences in the sentinel groups were: blood donors 4.5%, patients with fever 11.5%, anaemia patients 8.9%, urban STD patients 27.1%, and urban antenatal clinic attenders 12.1%. The crude prevalence in blood donors was 6.0%. It was concluded that blood donors who are relatives of blood acceptors were a representative sentinel group in this region, provided data were standardized for age, sex, and urban/non-urban location. Data from patients with fever markedly overestimated and data from antenatal clinic attenders underestimated population HIV-1 prevalence. Self-selection of blood donors may become more pronounced in the future, so this comparison should be repeated later or elsewhere if the opportunity occurs.

Chapter 5 presents a population based case-control study which was carried out to determine the relative and population attributable risk of HIV-1 infection for developing active tuberculosis (TB). Cases were 441 consecutively diagnosed patients with TB (all types), aged 15–54 years. Controls were taken from the population survey in Chapter 3, with a modified HIV-1 test strategy. The case detection rate of TB in those aged 15–54 years was 125/100,000 persons per year. The HIV-1 prevalence in cases was 23.0% in rural, 32.1% in roadside, and 54.1% in urban areas, while in controls these prevalences were 3.4%, 7.2% and 12.1%, respectively. The relative risk of HIV-1 infection for the development of active TB was estimated to be 8.3 (95% confidence interval 6.4–11.0). This risk varied little by sex or residence, but appeared to be more pronounced in the age group 25–34 years. The population attributable risk was 36/100,000 persons per year, implying that 29% of TB cases at present may be attributable to HIV-1 infection. It was concluded that HIV-1 infection is a major contributing factor to the increased case detection rate of TB observed over the past ten years in Mwanza Region.

Chapter 6 presents a case-control study which was carried out to determine the relative risk of HIV-1 infection for developing leprosy. Cases were 93 consecutively diagnosed patients with leprosy aged 15–54 years from Mwanza Region. Controls were taken from the population survey in Chapter 3, with a modified HIV-1 test strategy. The HIV-1 prevalence in cases was 10% in rural (7/72) and in roadside and urban areas (2/21), while in controls these prevalences were 3.4% and 9.9%, respectively. The relative risk of HIV-1 infection for the development of leprosy was estimated to be 2.2 (95% confidence interval (CI) 1.0–4.7; p=0.07). HIV-1 infection was significantly associated with multibacillary leprosy (odds ratio 4.6; 95% CI 1.3–13.2) but not with pauci-bacillary leprosy (odds ratio 1.4; 95% CI 0.4–3.8). The population etiological fraction for the development of multibacillary leprosy attributable to HIV-1 infection in this population can be estimated to be 13% (95% CI 4–23%). It was concluded that HIV-1 is a risk factor for the development of multibacillary leprosy. The impact of the HIV-1 epidemic on the incidence of leprosy has so far been limited, as HIV-1 occurs mainly in urban areas and leprosy in rural areas.

Chapter 7 describes the establishment of a cohort study of urban factory workers. First, the preparation of the study is presented with special attention to aspects such as: study objectives, selection of study site, assessing feasibility, obtaining approval, establish-ment of study clinic, development of data collection tools, informed consent for HIV testing, follow-up of non-attenders, and setting up procedures for data processing. In the second section, findings at intake from October 1991 to March 1992 are reported on risk factors for HIV-1 infection. HIV-1 prevalence was 91/926 (10%) in men and 36/217 (17%) in women. Statistically significant risk factors for HIV-1 infection in males were age group, region of birth, not being married for more than 5 years, being uncircum-cised, having had a genital ulcer in the past four months, and having received injections from medical staff in the past four months. HIV-1 incidence in this group was expected to be between 1% and 2% per year. It was concluded that a longitudinal study was needed to assess the importance of partner change. This cohort appeared to be suitable for such a study as HIV-1 incidence was expected to be fairly high, HIV-1 prevalence and risk factors were comparable to those of the general population, and cooperation of the factory workers was good.

Chapter 8 describes findings at intake from October 1991 to March 1992 on sexual partner change and condom use. Almost half of both men and women had had sexual intercourse by their 17th birthday. The period of premarital sex had an interquartile range of 2 to 10 years in men and 0 to 2.5 years in women. Having had sexual inter-course in the past month with more than one partner was reported by 22% of the men and 5% of the women. Factors associated with multiple partners in men were being born in or near Mwanza Region, having a low education and low income, and being married. Condoms had been used in the past month by 3% only, mainly with casual partners. Condom use in men was associated with being young, living in town, being born in Kagera Region, high education and high income, being circumcised, and having casual or steady (non-marital) partners. It was concluded that information, education, and communication (IEC) on sexual relationships and condom use should start at an early age, and include education at primary schools. Much sexual partner change appeared to occur through steady (non-marital) partnerships, indicating the need for IEC to be expanded beyond groups such as commercial sex workers and their clients.

In *Chapter 9* results are presented on HIV-1 incidence and HIV-1 associated mortality and morbidity after two years of follow-up. HIV-1 incidence was 1.2 (95% CI 0.7–1.8) per 100 person-years (pyr). Crude annual mortality was 4.9 per 100 pyr in those with and 0.3 in those without HIV-1 infection, giving an age- and sex-adjusted mortality ratio of 12.9 (95% CI 5.4–30.7). Of all deaths, 62% were attributable to HIV-1 infection. Clinical diagnoses in men associated with HIV-1 infection included fever, bacterial skin infections, tonsillitis/sore throat, diarrhoea and dysentery. HIV-1 infection in men was also associated with the prevalence and incidence of low body mass index, and with the presence and level of malaria parasitaemia, anaemia, and *E histolytica, G intestinalis, T hominis* and *S stercoralis* infection. In women, diarrhoea, herpes zoster, and genital discharge were associated with HIV-1 infection. It was concluded that HIV-1 was the major cause of death and substantially contributed to an increased morbidity in this adult population with an HIV-1 prevalence of 12% and an HIV-1 incidence of 1.2%. The number of HIV-1 seroconversions was only slightly larger than that of HIV-1-associated deaths, suggesting that the HIV-1 epidemic may have reached a steady-state level in this population.

In *Chapter 10* a general discussion is presented on the research results.

Epidemiologie van HIV-1-infectie in Mwanza-Regio, Tanzania: samenvatting

In dit proefschrift worden resultaten beschreven van onderzoek naar de epidemiologie van HIV-1-infectie bij volwassenen in Mwanza-Regio, Tanzania. Dit onderzoek werd uitgevoerd als onderdeel van het 'Tanzania-Netherlands Research Project on HIV Infection in Mwanza Region', waarvan de auteur de projectleider was.

In *Hoofdstuk 1* wordt een overzicht gegeven van de literatuur over de epidemiologie van HIV-1-infectie bij volwassenen in Afrika. In Afrika bestaat grote variatie in de incidentie van AIDS en in de prevalentie en incidentie van HIV-1-infectie. Tot nu toe is dit een veel groter probleem in Oost- dan in West-Afrika. De informatie over de incidentie en prevalentie van HIV-infectie en AIDS heeft beperkingen omdat de aangifte van gevallen van AIDS niet volledig is; groepen waarbij surveillance plaatsvindt niet altijd representatief zijn; en bij bevolkingsonderzoeken de dekkingsgraad niet volledig is. Risicofactoren voor heteroseksuele transmissie van HIV-1-infectie worden besproken, waaronder het wisselen van seksuele partners, het niet gebruiken van condooms, andere seksueel overdraagbare aandoeningen, de aanwezigheid van hoge concentraties virus in de met HIV-1-geïnfecteerde partner, seksuele technieken, besnijdenis van mannen, geslacht, leeftijd, woonplaats (stad-platteland), mobiliteit, and sociaal-economische status. Interventies voor het verminderen van heteroseksuele HIV-1-transmissie worden gepresenteerd, in het bijzonder programma's voor het bevorderen van (1) gedrags-verandering (vermindering van wisseling van seksuele partners), (2) condoomgebruik, en (3) vroege behandeling van seksueel overdraagbare aandoeningen. De huidige kennis over het natuurlijk verloop van HIV-1-infectie bij volwassenen in Afrika wordt besproken, in het bijzonder de incubatietijd, de met HIV-1 geassocieerde mortaliteit en morbiditeit, en met name de interactie van HIV-1 met tuberculose, lepra, en malaria.

Hoofdstuk 2 geeft achtergrondinformatie over Tanzania en Mwanza-Regio en beschrijft de ontwikkeling, voornaamste activiteiten en organisatie van het 'Tanzania-Netherlands Research Project on HIV infection in Mwanza Region'. Tanzania ligt in Oost-Afrika en heeft een laag inkomen per hoofd van de bevolking (BNP per capita $ 100). Mwanza-Regio ligt aan het Victoriameer en had in 1990 een bevolking van 1.981.000 mensen. De regio fungeert als een handelscentrum in Noordwest-Tanzania, waar handelsroutes naar Uganda, Kenya, Rwanda, Burundi en Dar es Salaam samenkomen.

De eerste gevallen van AIDS in Tanzania werden aangegeven in 1983. Als deel van de op gang gebrachte bestrijding van de HIV/AIDS-epidemie in Tanzania startte in 1990 het 'Tanzania-Netherlands Research Project on HIV infection in Mwanza Region'. Het project had als doel bij te dragen tot de ontwikkeling van aan de lokale omstandigheden aangepaste en effectieve methoden voor het verminderen van HIV-besmetting door middel van het uitvoeren van epidemiologisch, gedragswetenschappelijk en klinisch onderzoek en proefinterventies. In dit proefschrift worden resultaten van een deel van het epidemiologisch onderzoek gepresenteerd.

Hoofdstuk 3 beschrijft een bevolkingsonderzoek in Mwanza-Regio, dat werd uit-gevoerd in 1990-91 om de prevalentie van HIV-1-infectie bij volwassenen te bepalen en om de belangrijkste risicofactoren te identificeren. Van de volwassen bevolking op het platteland was 2,5% met HIV-1 geïnfecteerd, in de dorpen langs de doorgaande wegen 7,3%, en in de stad 11,8%. HIV-1 kwam 1,5 keer zo vaak voor bij vrouwen als bij mannen. HIV-1 kwam vooral voor bij vrouwen van 15–34 jaar en bij mannen van 25–44 jaar. HIV-1- infectie kwam in verhoogde mate voor bij mensen die gescheiden waren of weduwe/weduwnaar, meerdere seksuele partners hadden gehad in de afgelopen 5 jaar, antilichamen hadden tegen syfilis, genitale afscheiding of een genitaal zweertje gehad hadden, in Mwanza-Stad geweest waren, en injecties gekregen hadden in het afgelopen jaar. HIV-1 was niet geassocieerd met besnijdenis van mannen. Geconcludeerd wordt dat de resultaten verenigbaar zijn met verspreiding van HIV-1 infectie langs de door-gaande wegen.

In *Hoofdstuk 4* wordt de HIV-1-prevalentie in verschillende groepen waarin surveillance plaatsvindt in de leeftijdsgroep 15–54 jaar, vergeleken met die in de algemene bevol-king, om te bepalen of het extrapoleren van deze surveillance-gegevens valide is. De HIV-1- prevalentie in de regio, gestandaardiseerd voor leeftijd, geslacht en woonplaats, was 4,1% (3,1% buiten de stad en 11,4% in de stad). De gestandaardiseerde HIV-1-prevalentie binnen de groepen onder surveillance was: bloeddonoren 4,5%, patiënten met koorts 11,5%, anemie patiënten 8,9%, SOA patiënten in de stad 27,1% en bezoek-sters van prenatale zorg 12,1%. De ongestandaardiseerde prevalentie onder bloed-donoren was 6,0%. Geconcludeerd werd dat bloeddonoren die familie waren van de ontvangers van het gedoneerde bloed, een representatieve groep waren voor surveil-lance in Mwanza-Regio, indien data werden gestandaardiseerd voor leeftijd, geslacht en woongebied (stad/platteland). Data van patiënten met koorts gaven een duidelijke overschatting en die van bezoeksters van prenatale zorg een onderschatting van de HIV-1-prevalentie in de algemene bevolking. Zelfselectie van bloeddonoren zou in de toekomst kunnen toenemen, zodat deze studie later of elders herhaald zou moeten worden als de gelegenheid zich voordoet.

Hoofdstuk 5 presenteert een patiënt-controle-onderzoek dat werd uitgevoerd om het relatieve en populatie-attributieve risico te bepalen van HIV-1-infectie voor het ont-wikkelen van actieve tuberculose. Patiënten waren 441 achtereenvolgens gediagnos-tiseerde tuberculose-gevallen (alle localisaties), in de leeftijdsgroep 15–54 jaar. De controlegroep was samengesteld uit degenen die deel uitmaakten van het bevolkings-onderzoek in Hoofdstuk 3, met een modificatie van de wijze waarop de HIV-1-infectiestatus was bepaald. Het aantal gevallen met tuberculose in de leeftijdsgroep

15–54 jaar was 125 per 100.000 personen per jaar. De HIV-1-prevalentie onder patiënten was 23,0% op het platteland, 32,1% langs de doorgaande wegen, en 54,1% in de stad, terwijl in de controlegroep deze prevalenties respectievelijk 3,4%, 7,2% en 12,1% waren. Het relatieve risico van HIV-1-infectie voor het ontwikkelen van actieve tuberculose werd geschat op 8,3 (95% betrouwbaarheidsinterval 6,4–11,0). Dit risico varieerde weinig met geslacht of woonplaats, maar leek meer uitgesproken in de leeftijdsgroep 25–34 jaar. Het populatie-attributief risico was 36 per 100.000 personen per jaar, hetgeen inhoudt dat 29% van de gevallen van tuberculose toe te schrijven was aan HIV-1-infectie. Geconcludeerd werd dat HIV-1-infectie veel heeft bijgedragen aan het toenemen van het aantal per jaar gevonden gevallen van tuberculose over de afgelopen tien jaar in Mwanza-Regio.

Hoofdstuk 6 presenteert een patiënt-controle-onderzoek dat werd uitgevoerd om het relatieve risico te bepalen van HIV-1-infectie voor het ontwikkelen van lepra. Patiënten waren 93 achtereenvolgens gediagnostiseerde lepragevallen in de leeftijdsgroep 15–54 jaar. De controlegroep was samengesteld uit degenen die deel uitmaakten van het bevolkingsonderzoek in Hoofdstuk 3, met een modificatie van de wijze waarop HIV-1-infectie status was bepaald. De HIV-1-prevalentie bij leprapatienten was 10% op het platteland (7/72) en in de stad (2/21), terwijl in de controlegroepen de prevalentie respectievelijk 3,4%, en 9,9% was. Het relatieve risico van HIV-1-infectie voor het ontwikkelen van lepra werd geschat op 2,2 (95% betrouwbaarheidsinterval (BI) 1,0–4,7; p=0.07). HIV-1-infectie was significant geassocieerd met multibacillaire lepra (odds ratio 4,6; 95% BI 1,3–13,2), maar niet met paucibacillaire lepra (odds ratio 1,4; 95% BI 0,4–3,8). Het deel van de multibacillaire lepragevallen in deze populatie dat toe te schrijven is aan HIV-1-infectie kan geschat worden op 13% (95% BI 4–23%). Geconcludeerd werd dat HIV-1 een risicofactor is voor het ontwikkelen van multibacillaire lepra. De gevolgen van de HIV-1-epidemie op de incidentie van lepra is tot nu toe beperkt gebleven omdat HIV-1 vooral in de stad voorkomt en lepra vooral op het platteland.

Hoofdstuk 7 beschrijft het opzetten van een cohortstudie van fabrieksarbeiders. Eerst wordt de voorbereiding van de studie gepresenteerd, in het bijzonder: studiedoeleinden, het selecteren van de plaats van de studie, het inschatten van de haalbaarheid, het verkrijgen van goedkeuring, het opzetten van een studiekliniek, het ontwikkelen van onderzoeksinstrumenten, het verkrijgen van *informed consent* voor het testen op HIV-infectie, het opvolgen van deelnemers die niet of te laat komen, en het opzetten van procedures voor dataverwerking. In het tweede deel worden de bevindingen gerapporteerd bij intrede in het onderzoek van oktober 1991 tot maart 1992 met betrekking tot risicofactoren voor HIV-1-infectie. De HIV-1-prevalentie was 91/926 (10%) bij mannen en 36/217 (17%) in vrouwen. Statistisch significante risicofactoren voor HIV-1-infectie bij mannen waren leeftijd, geboorteregio, niet langer dan 5 jaar getrouwd zijn, niet besneden zijn, een genitaal zweertje gehad te hebben in de afgelopen 4 maanden, en injecties gekregen te hebben van een 'westerse' medische staf in de afgelopen 4 maanden. De verwachte HIV-1-incidentie bij deze groep werd geschat op 1% tot 2% per jaar. Geconcludeerd werd dat een longitudinaal onderzoek nodig was om de gevolgen van wisseling van seksuele partners vast te stellen. Het cohort fabrieksarbeiders leek geschikt te zijn voor een dergelijke studie omdat de HIV-1-incidentie verwacht werd vrij hoog te zijn, de prevalentie van en de risicofactoren voor HIV-1-infectie vergelijkbaar waren met die in de algemene bevolking, en de medewerking van de fabrieksarbeiders aan het onderzoek goed was.

Hoofdstuk 8 beschrijft de bevindingen bij intrede in het onderzoek van oktober 1991 tot maart 1992 met betrekking tot het wisselen van seksuele partners en gebruik van condooms. Bijna de helft van zowel mannen als vrouwen hadden seksueel contact gehad voor hun 17e jaar. De periode van seks voor het huwelijk had een 25e en 75e percentiel van respectievelijk 2 en 10 jaar bij mannen en 0 en 2,5 jaar bij vrouwen. Van de mannen zei 22% seksueel contact te hebben gehad met meer dan een partner in de afgelopen maand, van de vrouwen was dit 5%. Er was een statistisch significante associatie bij mannen tussen enerzijds het hebben van meer dan één seksuele partner in de afgelopen maand en anderzijds geboren zijn in Mwanza-Regio, een laag niveau hebben van opleiding en inkomen, en gehuwd zijn. Condooms waren in de afgelopen maand gebruikt door 3% van de mensen, vooral bij losse seksuele contacten. Condoomgebruik bij mannen was geassocieerd met jonge leeftijd, wonen in de stad, geboorte in Kagera-Regio, een hoog niveau van opleiding en inkomen, besneden zijn, en het hebben van losse en vaste (voor- of buitenhuwelijkse) seksuele partners. Geconcludeerd werd dat gezondheidsvoorlichting over seksuele relaties en condoomgebruik vroeg zou moeten beginnen, en gedeeltelijk moet plaatsvinden op de lagere school. Veel wisseling van seksuele partners leek plaats te hebben binnen 'vaste' (voor- of buitenhuwelijkse) relaties, zodat gezondheidsvoorlichting zich niet zou moeten beperken tot groepen zoals verleners van betaalde seks en hun klanten.

In *Hoofdstuk 9* worden resultaten gepresenteerd met betrekking tot HIV-1-incidentie en met HIV-1 geassocieerde mortaliteit en morbiditeit in de eerste twee jaar na het begin van de cohortstudie. De HIV-1-incidentie was 1,2 (95% BI 0,7–1,8) per 100 persoon-jaren (pjr). Het bruto jaarlijks sterftecijfer was 4,9 per 100 pjr bij degenen met en 0,3 bij degenen zonder HIV-1-infectie, resulterend in een (leeftijds- en geslachtsgestandaardiseerd) relatief sterfterisico van 12,9 (95% BI 5,4–30,7). Van alle sterftegevallen was 62% toe te schrijven aan HIV-1-infectie. De volgende klinische diagnoses bij mannen waren geassocieerd met HIV-1-infectie: koorts, bacteriële huidinfecties, tonsillitis/zere keel, diarree en dysenterie. HIV-1-infectie bij mannen was ook geassocieerd met de prevalentie en incidentie van een lage Quetelet-index, en met de aanwezigheid en het niveau van malaria parasitaemie, met anemie, en met *E histolytica*, *G intestinalis*, *T hominis* en *S stercoralis* infectie. Bij vrouwen waren diarree, herpes zoster en genitale afscheiding geassocieerd met HIV-1-infectie. Geconcludeerd werd dat HIV-1 de voornaamste doodsoorzaak was en aanzienlijk bijdroeg aan een toegenomen morbiditeit in deze volwassen bevolking met een HIV-1-prevalentie van 12% en een HIV-1-incidentie van 1,2%. Het aantal HIV-1-seroconversies was slechts iets groter dan het aantal sterftegevallen in HIV-1-geïnfecteerden, hetgeen zou kunnen betekenen dat de HIV-1-epidemie een stabiel niveau heeft bereikt in deze bevolking.

In *Hoofdstuk 10* worden de onderzoeksresultaten nader bediscussieerd.

Acknowledgements

As the studies described in this thesis were carried out by many collaborators I would like to start with thanking all who made a contribution. However, I would like to thank some by name, because of their particular importance to the success of these studies or this thesis.

There are two people I would like to mention from the period before I got involved with this project, as I still felt their influence: Godfrey Walker, my tutor at the London School of Hygiene and Tropical Medicine who shared his enthusiasm for public health in developing countries and supported me in my attempts to write clearly in scientific language; and Corlien Varkevisser, who was a very inspiring person to work with and gave me a taste of the potential of interdisciplinary research.

In 1989, when I was employed by the Royal Tropical Institute, my first assignment was to work on the proposal of what was to be the TANERA Project. I am very grateful to Lex Muller, who had the confidence in me to employ me at the Institute and give me this assignment.

The proposal, which had been partly developed when I came in, owed much to Daan Mulder, Joas Rugemalila, Johan Leeuwenburg, and Henri van Asten. Henri van Asten continued to contribute a lot to the project from his position in Dar es Salaam, and it was always a pleasure to see him there or in Mwanza. The final research proposals owed much to many people, but I would like to mention in particular Joas Rugemalila, Richard Hayes, and Angus Nicoll for their contributions to the population survey and validation of sentinel surveillance.

In the initial stages, in the middle of administrative and other confusion about the shape of a project document, three people were particularly supportive: Prof W L Kilama, who with quiet humour showed the relativity of administrative barriers, and who never lost sight of the importance of getting applied HIV/AIDS research in Mwanza off the ground; Charles Gerhardt, who was a good teacher regarding what was involved in management and administration and a great collaborator in working on the draft project document; and Dr Nyamuryekung'e, who was very helpful in always finding time to meet and being able to indicate in a very clear and pleasant way what was needed and what had gone wrong.

In Mwanza, it was a privilege to work with the Regional Medical Officers Mrs Kigadye, Dr Madukwa (Acting), Dr Massesa; Directors of NIMR Mwanza Dr Rugemalila and Dr Gabone; and Directors of BMC Dr Kigadye, Dr Makwani (Acting), and Dr Berege. I would like to thank in particular Drs Massesa, Gabone, Makwani, and Berege, who made a success of the project management committee and who were extremely supportive in times of difficulty.

Of the colleagues in Mwanza I would like to thank first of all Longin Barongo, who was my host and counterpart from the very first days. He was a very pleasant colleague to work with and played a vital role in ensuring the project activities were known and acceptable to all those who mattered: local government, party, and trade union officials, health staff, and the population concerned. He was a good partner, with whom discussions on scientific plans were always lively and interesting. I also very much appreciated his willingness to share his knowledge of Tanzanian society.

I am also grateful to the other scientific staff of the epidemiological research team and cannot do justice to their major contributions in the few sentences that follow. Kesheni Senkoro was vital in keeping data processing under control; he worked with the dedication needed for quality work and always managed to stay in good humour. James Newell made the most of his part-time availability and made major contributions to data analysis; he was also very important in providing constructive criticism of draft papers. Arnoud Klokke was essential in being extremely competent and conscientious in carrying out the HIV laboratory work; his interest in new laboratory techniques was stimulating. John Changalucha was extremely supportive in setting up procedures for field work, and in the establishment of new microbiological techniques in the laboratory. Ties Boerma, my successor in Mwanza, I thank for his support in sending additional information where needed and for his critical comments on drafts. I was glad to hand over this task to such a capable successor.

The commitment of all staff involved in field work was very encouraging. I would like to mention in particular the staff who were involved right from the start of the factory cohort study: Yusuf Kumogola, Peter Ignas, Victoria Hillu, Agatha Joachim, Milalu Ndege, Dr Mutungi, Dr Mwita, Dr Ngalula, Dr Songora, Mrs Makwani, Mr Chande, Mr Bulaya, Mr Ndokeji, Mr Nditi, Mrs Barongo, and Mrs Masalu. The work would literally have come to a stand-still without Mr S Chongela and Justin Mtungi. I am particularly grateful to Mtungi who was not only an excellent, hard working, and punctual driver, but also an 'executive officer' and a friend of the family.

I would also like to express my gratitude for the cooperation and hospitality we experienced from the people of Mwanza Region when we carried out the population survey. The cooperation and support of the workers, the management, and trade union of the textile factory was very much appreciated. I am particularly grateful for the support of Mr Marwa, General Manager, and Mr Shungu, Manpower Development and Administrative Manager. Very active day-to-day support was given by Mr Rwegoshora and Mr Kajenge.

Essential laboratory work and data processing were done by many, including in the laboratory Mr Shija, Ms Shushu, and Mr Mngara, and in the statistical unit Ms Jasmine Rwenza and Ms Z Balinda. I am very greatful to Ms Grace Panga (personal secretary), the accounts section (head: Mr D Komba), and administration (heads: Mr B Kamugisha, thereafter Mr G Mwenda) of NIMR Mwanza for their pleasant and effective support to project administration.

Continuous support was given by the Managers of the National AIDS Control Programme Dr K M Nyamuryekung'e and Dr R O Swai; the National Institute for

Medical Research Headquarters, in particular Prof W L Kilama and Dr J Rugemalila; the Royal Netherlands Embassy, in particular Maarten Brouwer, Arnold van Hengel, Bob Hensen and Thomas van der Heijden; and the Ministry of Foreign Affairs/DGIS/ DST/SO, in particular Martin de la Bey and Hans Moerkerk. Collaboration was very fruitful with Heiner Grosskurth, Project Manager of the African Medical and Research Foundation (AMREF), and Jacques van den Broek, Regional Tuberculosis/Leprosy Coordinator.

I would like to thank the following consultants to the epidemiological studies: Japheth Killewo, Lex Muller, Johan Velema, Roel Coutinho, and Walter Deville. They came as experts but left as friends, and their support was much appreciated.

Roel Coutinho and Lex Muller I would like to thank also for being extremely supportive in their supervision during the writing of this thesis: they clearly pointed out the major issues, and always were very positive and constructive in discussions with an excellent atmosphere. I thank Prof dr J Huisman, Prof dr J van der Noordaa, Prof dr J P Tijssen, and Dr C Varkevisser too, for being prepared to be members of the 'promotie-commissie'.

I also thank the Royal Tropical Institute for allowing me the time needed to complete this thesis.

Finally, I would like to express my gratitude to Jennechien for supporting me in writing this thesis, reading and criticizing drafts, and being a great support when times were difficult. I am also grateful for her willingness to come with me to far away places and thereby delay her settling in as a general practitioner. Finally, I thank Jennechien, Joris and Hanneke for their tolerance as I worked on the computer and was distracted while producing this thesis. I very much appreciate their continuous support.